Endorsements

'With a heart of gold and a passion for holistic health, the pioneer of aromatherapy Dr Blossom Kochhar believes that what you put on your face, you should be able to eat! *The Glow Getter's Guide to Everyday Skincare* is a treasure trove of natural beauty and self-care tips emanating from four decades of dedicated practice.

True to her name, Blossom glows with goodness and has dedicated her life's work to spreading the radiance of health and well-being naturally. Just meeting her is to feel rejuvenated! This book is not just about looking good, but about feeling good as well. With advice on the importance of inner care, stress relief, mindfulness, and maintaining a healthy lifestyle, *The Glow Getter's Guide to Everyday Skincare* offers easy-to-follow DIY recipes to nourish you inside out. Whether you are an expert beauty enthusiast or just starting on your beauty trail, this book must be added to your self-care library.'

Vinita Dawra Nangia
Columnist, Author, and Executive Editor at The Times Group

'This book is a treasure trove of holistic secrets to radiant skin and hair and overall well-being. Dr Blossom Kochhar shares invaluable insights and practical advice on time-tested desi *nuskhas*. Whether you're just starting your skincare journey or are already an enthusiast, this comprehensive guide by Dr Kochhar is a must-have for all.'

Rajshri Deshpande
Actor and Social Worker

THE GLOW GETTER'S GUIDE TO EVERYDAY SKINCARE

Dr Blossom Kochhar

HAY HOUSE INDIA
New Delhi • London • Sydney
Carlsbad, California • New York City

Hay House Publishers (India) Pvt Ltd
Muskaan Complex, Plot No. 3, B-2, Vasant Kunj, New Delhi – 110070, India

Hay House LLC, P.O. Box 5100, Carlsbad, CA 92018-5100, USA
Hay House UK Ltd, The Sixth Floor, Watson House, 54 Baker Street, London W1U 7BU, UK
Hay House Australia Publishing Pty Ltd, 18/36 Ralph St., Alexandria NSW 2015, Australia

Email: contact@hayhouse.co.in
Website: www.hayhouse.co.in

First published by Hay House India, 2024
10 9 8 7 6 5 4 3 2 1

ISBN 978-81-97222-83-2
ISBN 978-81-97222-86-3 (Ebook)

Printed at Replika Press Pvt Ltd

FSC
www.fsc.org
MIX
Paper | Supporting responsible forestry
FSC™ C016779

Hay House is committed to a sustainable future for our business, our readers and our planet. This book is made from Forest Stewardship Council® certified paper.

To my daughter, Samantha,
and my grandson, Aryman,
for being my pillars of strength

Contents

III
Nourishing Your Locks

IV
Beauty from Within

Author's Note

Self-care is an important aspect of self-love, and we all need to invest time in ourselves. However, in today's fast-paced and stressed world, beauty has been reduced to simply reaching for a jar of cosmetics, which we buy online or from a store counter. But that isn't always beneficial. We are meticulous about what we eat and consider its impact on us. But have you ever thought about the fact that our skin is the body's largest organ, constantly breathing and living? What we put on it enters our body and can have adverse effects as well. I've always maintained that 'what you put on your face, you should be able to eat,' and vice versa. So, take some time out for wholesome, homemade beauty indulgence.

I've always been in favour of utilising ingredients from your kitchen shelf for beauty purposes. This book is an attempt to revive the DIY recipes that were likely used by your grandmother.

One common question is, 'Where is the time to do DIY?' I believe you should carve out a little time, perhaps, once or twice a week or whenever you need to pamper yourself and indulge in a DIY beauty recipe. It will benefit you tremendously because that is the time you are dedicating to self-care.

The book contains numerous recipes for skin, hair, and body care. I invite you to try these recipes, and I'm sure you will enjoy making and using them as much as I enjoyed sharing them with you.

Additionally, there are a few pointers here on inner beauty because beauty is holistic and is greatly influenced by a balanced body, mind, and emotions. Caring for your skin, hair, and body goes beyond mere beauty; it also has a significant impact on your health and emotions. Even the wise have said that we must look after our bodies, for this is where the divine resides.

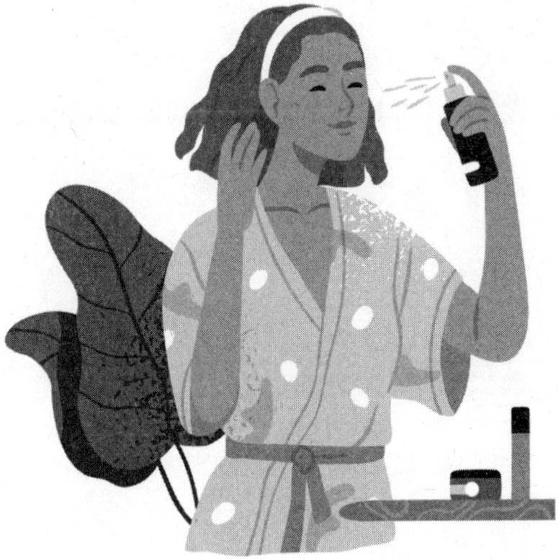

I
FACIAL CARE

1
All about Skin

Good skincare begins from day one. In my career, spanning over four decades, I have always imparted one simple advice for good skin—regular and consistent skincare. However, it is important to first understand your skin, its structure, and functions to follow an effective day-to-day skincare regime and to deal with common skin problems.

What does healthy skin entail? Healthy and bright skin is free from blemishes—like scars—is soft and plump, hydrated, smooth and glowing (reflecting light and with clear visibility of the inner skin), supple, firm, wrinkle-free (toned, elastic and collagen enriched) and having no visible acne or allergy (unsusceptible to infection).

Our skin comprises three layers—the epidermis, the dermis, and the hypodermis. All these layers perform different functions.

The Epidermis

The outer layer, the epidermis, is the part that we see and touch. It is composed of flattened keratinocytes (also known as dead horny cells) formed by the protein keratin and a basal cell layer beneath it where the new cells are manufactured. The new cells move to the surface where they die and are then exfoliated. The epidermis has no blood vessels or nerves.

The Dermis

The dermis is commonly known as the true skin and is the thick layers below the epidermis. It comprises connective tissues, which include collagen, protein, and elastic fibres (elastic-type protein) that form a valuable support system for the skin. It is in this layer that most of the skin's ageing process takes place—the sweat glands, the oil glands, the nerve endings and receptors, blood vessels, arrector pili muscles (APM), and a major portion of hair follicles are in the dermis. Melanin cells, which are responsible for freckles and darkening of the skin in sunlight, are also present in the dermis.

The Hypodermis

The hypodermis or sub-dermis is a subcutaneous tissue or fatty layer situated below the dermis. It influences the quality of our skin's appearance. A dramatic fat loss can cause the skin to sag and high fat or water retention in the skin's tissue can make it stretch, creating dimples. The hypodermis acts as the skin's cushion, absorbing shock to protect the bones and help support delicate structures, such as blood vessels, nerve endings, and hair bulbs. This layer contours and shapes the body, acting as an emergency reservoir of food and water.

Understanding Skin Functions

My clients are usually surprised when I explain that skin does more than just protect. Apart from protecting the internal organs, the skin performs six other significant functions.

1. Detoxification: The skin eliminates toxic waste products and water from the body. If these are not removed

properly, it may lead to a sallow and dull complexion, swelling throughout the body, and aggravation of acne.

2. Regulation: The skin helps regulate the body temperature. It maintains the internal temperature according to the external environment.
3. Sensation: All the sensations we feel in our body are processed through our skin. The nerve endings beneath the skin make us aware of heat, cold, pain, and pleasure, allowing us to react accordingly.
4. Hydration: Hydration helps maintain the skin's moisture level by releasing perspiration. Moreover, the oily sebaceous matter acts as the skin's best lubricant.
5. Absorption: The skin acts as a carrier of substances to the body, permitting certain substances to pass through its tissues. This is why oils, creams, and moisturisers are applied through the skin.
6. Respiration: The skin also breathes, albeit in a limited capacity compared to the lungs. It can absorb oxygen and release carbon dioxide and other unwanted gases.

Skincare Hacks

Normally, healthy skin would require minimal attention to be spent for its care in terms of time and effort. However, inadequate or improper care can run down and ruin healthy and happy skin. Thus, it is crucial to follow a regular and customised skincare routine that addresses your concerns and provides you with a natural glow.

Skin is a canvas that reflects your internal system as well as your mental health. If you want your skin to look radiant and healthy, there are a few rules that you need to follow. Internal care requires a sensible diet, plenty of water intake, adequate sleep, moderate exercise, and a calm disposition, which, in turn, can make your skin look healthy and luminous.

Move Your Body

Oxygen is vital to your skin, and blood cells carrying both oxygen and nourishment circulate to every part of your body, including your skin. If you continuously breathe in stagnant, stale air, you cannot expect your skin to look pink and glowing with good health. Deep breathing exercises are a beauty treatment in themselves, especially when you fill your lungs with pure, fresh air.

A brisk half-an-hour walk every day can be as beneficial as an expensive facial, especially if you are relaxed and dressed for the walk, and, above all, enjoying the walk. You will return home with a glow on your cheeks, and a sparkle in your eyes, and your skin will tingle with vitality. Exercise revs up the circulation of oxygen to the skin.

Emotions

Your skin is an accurate barometer of your feelings. It is important to be mentally fit and happy to have healthy and glowing skin. Fits of temper or bouts of depression may result in outbreaks of blemishes or rashes. Next time you lose your temper, count to ten.

Diet

Our skin reflects what we eat and drink. Eating the right balance of foods will provide your skin with the vital nutrients it needs to stay healthy. Foods that promote healthy skin include fruit and vegetables, lean meat, dairy products, and whole-grain breads and cereals. However, be moderate in your intake of sweets, chocolate, starches, greasy foods, and food to which you may be sensitive. If you break out in hives the day after eating fish or prawns, or if you develop bumps after indulging in chocolate, you know which foods to restrict in your diet. Drinking six glasses of water a day, along with additional liquids in the form of juices, green tea, and milk, will also contribute to healthy skin.

Detoxification

Establish regular habits to flush waste from your body. Retained toxins in your body may show up as dull skin colour, dark circles under the eyes, or skin blemishes. Eating a couple of figs or dates each day can help facilitate daily waste disposal. An excellent remedy for constipation is an early morning drink of lemon juice and water, or a teaspoon of malt vinegar and a tablespoon of honey stirred into a glass of hot water. Another trick is to soak the dates overnight in a cup of water. In the morning, mash the dates in the water and drink it before your morning tea.

Sleep

Your skin rejuvenates itself while you sleep; thus, sleeping eight to ten hours at night is beneficial. Additionally, well-rested skin is more receptive to skincare products, making them more effective.

Build a Skincare Regimen

I have often been asked this question: 'Your skin looks great. What is the secret?' There's no secret. However, my skincare routine revolves around the CTM routine—cleansing, toning, moisturising—which I follow twice a day. Additionally, I use face oils, serums, night creams, and gel-based face packs. The usage of these products varies from one skin type to another.

Cleansing: This is the most important aspect of skincare. It removes stale make-up, cleans the skin pores, and exfoliates the dead cells that can cause blockages on the skin's surface. I prefer a cream cleanser since my skin is dry. At night, I do a double cleanse to ensure all make-up, dirt, and grime are removed completely.

Toning: Cleansing should be followed by toning. A splash of toner works wonders for all skin types. It helps in stimulating the skin, tightening pores, and invigorating blood circulation. However, until not too long ago, it was believed that toning is only necessary for oily skin. I recommend toning for all skin types but always remember to use a non-alcoholic toner.

Moisturising: Moisturising is an important step in any daily skincare routine. It keeps the skin hydrated.

Oiling/Serum: Conditioning restores the skin's acid balance, nourishes the skin, and corrects imbalances. Conditioning includes skin oils and night creams. Essential oils can also work wonders for your skin; they are neither oily nor greasy and can be used to balance every skin type. Different skin types require different essential oils to balance and nourish the skin.

In the following chapters, we will explore how to care for each skin type and address different concerns according to the seasons, helping you achieve that natural and healthy glow.

2

Care for Every Skin Type

Every individual has a unique skin type, and this can be broadly characterised into three types—oily, dry, and combination. To take proper care of your skin, it's essential to understand your skin type. If your skin is oily, you'll need products that help control excess oil. If it's dry, look for products that provide extra hydration and moisture. If your skin is a combination of both, you'll need to balance the needs of the dry and oily areas. By using the right skincare products for your skin type, you can achieve healthier and more radiant skin, which will improve your overall complexion.

Know Your Skin Type

To understand your skin type, you need a few strips of tissue paper or paper napkins. In the morning, before washing your face, gently rub the strips across your forehead, nose, chin, and cheeks. The strips could either become stained with grease or stay clear and clean.

a. If all the strips are greasy, including the one used on the cheek, and the stains are large, you have extremely oily skin.
b. If the strips used on the forehead, nose, and chin are greasy whereas the ones used on the cheeks are clean, you have a combination skin.

c. If all the strips are clean, with no stains at all, you have dry skin.

Through the strip-test method, one can find out their skin type as well as which parts of the face are excessively oily or dry. Now, we'll explore in detail the different skin types and how to care for your skin accordingly.

Oily Skin

Oily skin has a shiny appearance, often with large, visible pores. Individuals with this skin type may experience blackheads and whiteheads in different areas of their face.

My clients often bring their adolescents to me who are worried about their oily skin and the woes that accompany it. The oiliness is largely caused due to the over-activity of the sebaceous glands and the overproduction of oil. If a proper cleansing routine is not followed, the condition can get worse. The nervous and hormonal irregularities that occur in our bodies are responsible for the over-activity of the oil glands.

Oily skin looks greasy and unclean and with visibly enlarged pores. Over time, blockages of grime, stale make-up, and dead cells appear in the skin pores, resulting in the formation of whiteheads and blackheads. The excessive oiliness causes a sallow, yellow complexion and thick, coarse skin texture. The make-up, too, changes and disappears easily.

Taking care of oily skin is especially challenging and cumbersome. To treat oily skin, it is important to carry out a meticulous cleansing routine, sloughing off the dead cells, and removal of make-up, excess oil, and grime embedded in the pores.

This involves washing the face and neck at least twice a day with a mild, medicated face wash. Avoid using creamy and fat-enriched cleansers and creams. Concentrate especially on the forehead, nose, and chin area by thoroughly massaging the lather, then rinse your face with cold water.

Furthermore, after cleansing your skin, use a non-alcoholic toner to tone and tighten enlarged pores. If your skin feels taut and dry afterwards, apply a gel-based moisturiser that won't clog the pores or irritate your skin.

Types of Oily Skin

There are essentially two types of oily skin. Understanding the kind of oily skin you have can help you tailor your skincare routine accordingly to manage oil production and maintain healthy, balanced skin.

Classic Oily Skin

Most of my clients come for consultation when their skin appears to be shiny and feels greasy, especially in the T-zone—forehead, nose, and chin areas. This is due to the overproduction of sebum (skin oil) by the sebaceous glands. Their skin is prone to enlarged pores, blackheads, and acne breakouts.

I advise them to use a gentle, foaming cleanser to control oil without excessively drying out the skin. I also suggest using a face wash that consists of BHAs (beta hydroxy acid). It's essential to use all gel-based products, including moisturisers, and a non-alcoholic toner to avoid clogging the pores. Furthermore, rose water and apple cider vinegar can be beneficial. Avoid using oil-based products. Use minimal make-up and a soothing sunscreen gel every day since you are exfoliating regularly.

Oily Skin with Sensitivity

Many of my clients come to me with highly sensitive oily skin that reacts to all skincare products, causing redness, irritation, and inflammation.

I advise them to clean their skin with yoghurt only if they are not allergic to lactic acid. I suggest using fragrance-free and hypoallergenic skincare products. They can apply aloe vera gel with 1–2 drops of lavender essential oil all over the skin, which acts as a moisturiser. I advise them to tone their skin with pure rose water. Lastly, they should store their skincare items in the fridge to avoid skin irritation caused by heat.

Oily Skin: Causes and Triggers

1. Hormonal changes, such as puberty, pregnancy, or menstrual cycles can lead to oily skin because of overactive sebaceous glands.
2. Your genetic make-up can also cause oily skin tendencies.
3. Although the relationship between diet and oily skin is complex and varies from person to person, it is best to avoid greasy or fried foods or food rich in iodine, like seafood, along with chocolates as much as possible. It's best to consume them in moderation.
4. Using skincare products that are too harsh or drying can disrupt the skin's natural balance, prompting it to produce more oil to compensate.
5. Hot and humid weather can trigger excess oil production.
6. High-stress levels can stimulate the body to release cortisol, which, in turn, increases oil production.

7. Ironically, excessive cleansing can strip away too much oil, causing the skin to produce more to compensate.

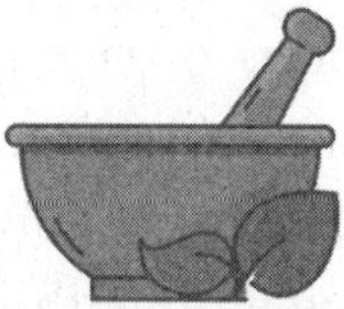

Nourishing DIY Recipes for Oily Skin

There are plenty of products in the market for oily skin. It is a tedious process to experiment and find out which product suits you the best. However, your kitchen, too, has several useful natural ingredients that can help deal with the issue. Here are some DIY recipes that can aid in making your skin look bright and healthy.

Cleansing

Recipe 1: Use a face wash or a cleanser meant for oily skin. Another great cleanser for oily skin is applying a mix of plain yoghurt with a little salt. Gently massage it on your face before washing it off.

Recipe 2: Take one teaspoon of aloe vera gel and add two drops of tea tree oil. Use this as a cleanser and wash it off with cold water.

Scrubbing

Recipe 1: Mix 1/4 cup of Multani mitti (fuller's earth), 1/4 cup of dried orange peel powder, and 2 tablespoons of sandalwood powder or oatmeal. Store this mixture in a container in your bathroom. Mix one teaspoon of the mixture with water and work it into the skin, then rinse it with warm water. Make sure to use it every other day.

Recipe 2: Take 2 teaspoons of rice powder and mix it with enough yoghurt to form a paste. Squeeze 2–3 drops of lemon juice. Gently work this paste into your skin and leave it on for 10 minutes before rinsing it off with warm water. You can use this every alternate day.

Recipe 3: Take green tea leaves from a used tea bag. Add 1/2 teaspoon of glycerine and 1 teaspoon of powdered sugar. Apply the mixture on your face and gently work it in. Rinse it off after 10 minutes.

Toning

Recipe 1: Mix cucumber juice with rose water, and keep a bottle of this toner handy for frequent use during the day. It makes for an excellent toner!

Recipe 2: Take 5–6 drops of apple cider vinegar and add 1 tablespoon of rose water to it. Use this concoction to splash on your face.

Masks

Recipe 1: Mix 1/4 cup of Multani mitti with some tomato pulp and yoghurt. Apply and leave it on the face for 15–20 minutes before rinsing it off with water. Use this mask at least twice a week.

Recipe 2: Crush 10 mint leaves and mix it with 2 teaspoons of yoghurt and one teaspoon of cucumber juice. Also, add one drop of peppermint essential oil. Apply it on your face and wash it off after 15 minutes.

Recipe 3: Make a paste of 1 beaten egg white, 1 tablespoon of yoghurt, and 1 tablespoon of Multani mitti. Then, add 1 drop of tea tree essential oil and 1 drop of patchouli essential oil. Apply this mixture to your face and leave it on until it dries. Rinse it off with clear water. Use this toning mask at least twice a week.

Dos for Oily Skin

1. Do Cleanse Regularly: Wash your face twice daily with a gentle, sulphate-free cleanser to remove excess oil, dirt, and impurities without over-drying your skin.
2. Do Use Oil-Free or Non-Comedogenic Products: Choose skincare products, including moisturisers and sunscreens, that are labelled 'oil-free' or 'non-comedogenic' to avoid clogging your pores.
3. Do Exfoliate: Use a BHA exfoliant 2–3 times a week to help unclog pores, reduce blackheads, and improve skin texture.
4. Do Apply a Lightweight Moisturiser: Even oily skin needs hydration. Choose a lightweight, gel-based moisturiser to keep your skin's moisture balance in check.
5. Do Use Sunscreen Daily: Apply a broad-spectrum sunscreen with an SPF of 30 or higher every

morning, regardless of the weather, to protect your skin from sun damage.

6. Do Blot Excess Oil: Carry blotting papers or oil-absorbing sheets to gently blot away excess oil during the day without disturbing your make-up.
7. Do Maintain a Balanced Diet: Consume a balanced diet rich in fruits, vegetables, and whole grains, while minimising greasy and fried foods.
8. Do Stay Hydrated: Drink plenty of water throughout the day to keep your body and skin well-hydrated.
9. Do Manage Stress: High stress levels can trigger increased oil production. Practise stress-management techniques such as yoga, meditation, or deep breathing exercises.
10. Do Consult a Dermatologist: If you have persistent or severe oily skin concerns, seek advice from a dermatologist for personalised skincare recommendations and treatments.

Don'ts for Oily Skin

1. Don't Over-Cleanse: Avoid excessive cleansing or using harsh, abrasive scrubs, as this can strip the skin of its natural oils and lead to a rebound in oil production.
2. Don't Use Harsh Products: Steer clear of skincare products that contain alcohol, strong astringents,

or high levels of fragrances, as they can irritate and dry out the skin.

3. Don't Skip Moisturiser: Skipping moisturiser can make oily skin worse. Always use a lightweight, non-comedogenic moisturiser to maintain hydration.
4. Don't Touch Your Face: Refrain from touching your face with your hands, as this can transfer dirt and bacteria, exacerbating breakouts.
5. Don't Pick or Squeeze Spots: Avoid picking, squeezing, or popping spots, as this can lead to scarring and increased oil production.
6. Don't Overload on Make-up: Applying too much make-up can clog pores and make oily skin appear more pronounced. Use oil-free or mineral make-up and avoid heavy foundations.
7. Don't Skip Sunscreen: Never skip sunscreen, even if you believe it makes your skin feel oilier. Sunscreen is crucial for preventing sun damage and premature ageing.
8. Don't Use Hot Water: Avoid scalding hot water when cleansing your face or showering, as it can strip the skin of its natural oils. Use lukewarm water instead.
9. Don't Use Bar Soap: Bar soap is often too harsh for oily skin and can disrupt its pH balance. Stick to a gentle liquid cleanser.

10. Don't Forget to Adjust for Seasonal Changes: Your skincare routine may need adjustments depending on the season and weather conditions. Be flexible in your approach to address changing needs.

Dry Skin

I particularly empathise with dry skin people since my skin tends to get dry as well. If you have dry skin, you first need to figure out which type of dryness you have. There are mainly two different dry skin conditions—the oil-dry and the moisture-dry. The oil-dry skin is sensitive and often has flaky patches with no visible pores. It tends to age and wrinkle prematurely unless carefully cared for. This kind of dryness is caused by the sluggish activity of the oil glands, resulting in inadequate oil secretion and insufficient skin lubrication. Apart from the improper functioning of the sebaceous glands, factors such as anxiety, improper diet, using the wrong cosmetics, strong soaps, overexposure to the sun, and harsh winds can aggravate dryness.

On the other hand, the moisture-dry skin has a fine texture. Its appearance is taut and dry with a tendency to chap easily. Even at an early age, it may show fine lines around the eyes and mouth. This kind of dryness is caused by the inadequate functioning of the sweat glands and internal dehydration. Excessive exposure to the sun and wind can worsen dryness. To combat this sort of dryness, it is highly recommended to increase your intake of liquids and use moisturisers. These simple steps can be extremely helpful in keeping your skin hydrated and healthy.

Types of Dry Skin

Dry skin can manifest in various ways and may be caused by multiple factors. There are different types of dry skin:

Dehydrated Skin

Dehydrated skin is a temporary condition often caused by external factors like weather, harsh skincare products, or lack of proper hydration. Symptoms may include tightness, flakiness, and a dull complexion.

Individuals with dehydrated skin need to apply moisturisers or creams on damp skin. They should use a mild toner, such as a rose water spray, regularly. Regularly using a Hyaluronic acid serum before applying moisturiser can aid in keeping the skin plump.

Xerotic Skin

Xerotic skin is a chronic condition that leads to extremely dry or rough skin and typically occurs due to ageing. It's characterised by rough, scaly patches, which are more common in older adults. Individuals with this kind of skin cannot use any soap or face washes. So, I always recommend they apply a cold cream to cleanse their skin, which needs to be applied all over the body instead of soap. They can then wipe it off with a rough towel. Make sure to avoid using hot water.

Asteatotic Skin

Asteatotic skin is characterised by fine cracks and a 'crazy-paving' pattern. It's often linked to very low humidity levels and is more prevalent in winter months. For such skin, I recommend slugging. Slugging involves following your skincare routine for dry skin and then applying a layer of Vaseline to keep the moisture intact. This process should be included in your nighttime routine. However, a very thin layer of Vaseline can be used in the daytime.

Furthermore, keep a good quality humidifier at home to add moisture to the indoor environment. Use a mild, cream-based cleanser to avoid further dryness, followed by a thick, cream-based moisturiser to create a protective barrier. Avoid taking long, hot showers, and consider incorporating oatmeal masks to soothe irritation.

Consult a dermatologist for skin conditions like eczema and psoriasis that require long-term treatments.

Dry Skin: Causes and Triggers

1. Harsh weather conditions, such as cold winters or hot, dry summers, can strip the skin of its natural moisture and lead to excessive dryness.
2. Indulging in scalding hot showers and baths may be relaxing, but they can also remove the skin's natural oils, leaving it parched.
3. Certain skincare products, especially those containing alcohol or harsh chemicals, can disrupt the skin's barrier function, contributing to dryness.
4. As we age, our skin naturally loses moisture and becomes less efficient at retaining water, leading to drier skin.
5. Conditions like eczema, psoriasis, and thyroid disorders can exacerbate dry skin, requiring specialised care.

6. A diet lacking in essential fatty acids and water can leave your skin thirsty for nourishment.

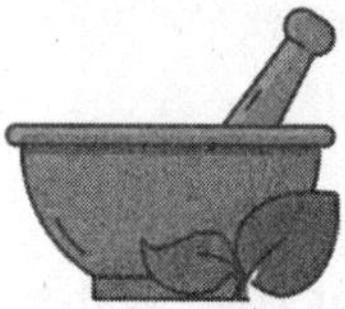

Nourishing DIY Recipes for Dry Skin

Cleanser

Recipe 1: Add a dash of turmeric to some milk and use it as a cleanser.

Recipe 2: Warm a cup of milk, add 1 teaspoon of glycerine and 1/4 teaspoon of bicarbonate of soda. Stir the mixture until it dissolves completely, and then apply it as a cleanser.

Mild Scrub

Recipe 1: Take 1 tablespoon of fresh cream, and some powdered almonds, mix and apply it on your face. Gently scrub and rinse it off with lukewarm water. Use this only once a week.

Recipe 2: In 1 tablespoon of cream, add 1 teaspoon of oatmeal powder and a pinch of turmeric. Mix and gently scrub your face with it. Use this twice a week.

Toner

Recipe 1: Rose water is an excellent toner for dry skin. You can use it twice a day.

Recipe 2: Add 5–6 drops of Hyaluronic acid serum to 1 tablespoon of rose water and mix it nicely. Keep it handy and use it as a toner.

Moisturiser

Recipe 1: Mix 3/4 cup of rose water, 1/4 cup of glycerine, 1 teaspoon of vinegar, and 1/4 teaspoon of honey. Store this mixture in a bottle. Use it regularly after cleansing and toning your face.

Recipe 2: Create your face oil by blending 3 drops of sandalwood oil, 1 tablespoon of almond oil, and 3 drops of castor oil. Apply it on your face and remove any excess with a tissue after 5 minutes.

Nourishing Mask

Recipe 1: Mash a banana and beat in a teaspoon of vegetable oil. If you are not allergic, add 1 teaspoon of honey to the mix. Apply the mask to your face and leave it for 20 minutes before rinsing it off. Use it once a week to hydrate your skin.

Recipe 2: Other fruits that can be used for dry skin are melons and avocadoes. Mash the fruit of your choice, add a drop of sandalwood oil to it and apply the mixture on your face. Once it dries, wash it off with warm water.

Dos for Dry Skin

1. Do Keep Hydrated: Drink plenty of water to keep your body and skin well-hydrated from the inside.

2. Do Cleanse Gently: Use a mild, hydrating cleanser that won't strip off the natural oils.
3. Do Moisturise: Apply a moisturiser with ingredients like hyaluronic acid, glycerine, or ceramides to lock in moisture.
4. Do Protect Yourself from the Sun: Always wear sunscreen to shield your skin from UV damage, which can worsen dryness.
5. Do Apply DIY Masks: Incorporate hydrating DIY masks into your skincare routine, tailored to your specific type of dry skin.
6. Do Go for Specialised Treatments: Depending on the severity of your dry skin, consider professional treatments like microneedling, microdermabrasion, or chemical peels under expert guidance.

Don'ts for Dry Skin

1. Don't Use Hot Water: Avoid hot showers or baths, as they can dehydrate the skin by stripping off natural oils.
2. Don't Apply Harsh Products: Steer clear of skincare products containing alcohol, fragrances, or harsh chemicals.
3. Don't Over-exfoliate: Limit exfoliation to prevent further dryness. Once or twice a week is usually sufficient.

4. Don't Pick: Refrain from picking at dry patches of skin or using abrasive scrubs as this can damage your already compromised skin barrier.
5. Don't Ignore Medical Conditions: If your dry skin is due to an underlying medical condition, consult a dermatologist for proper diagnosis and care.

Combination Skin

As the name suggests, combination skin is partly dry and partly oily skin. Usually, the central part of the face, also known as the T-zone—the forehead, nose, chin—and certain areas of the cheeks look greasy, while other parts appear dry.

This kind of skin requires care that helps the conditions part-oily and part-dry conditions. Maintaining such skin type can be especially challenging because of climate or stress. I advise my clients to cleanse their skin twice a day with a mild cleanser. I have also found that rose water is the ideal toner for this kind of skin.

For moisturising and conditioning, I recommend using two face oils. For dry areas, apply a mixture of 1 tablespoon of almond oil with 2 drops of sandalwood oil. To combat oiliness, apply a mixture of 2 drops of tea tree oil in aloe vera gel.

Lastly, use a hot towel as a compress on your entire face.

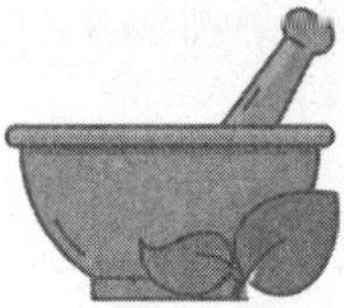

Nourishing DIY Recipes for Combination Skin

Recipe 1: Take a small piece of papaya and mash it. Add a squeeze of lemon to it. Mix properly and apply it on oily areas.

Recipe 2: Add 1/2 teaspoon of milk powder and 2 drops of sandalwood to some mashed papaya. Apply this mixture to dry areas.

Additional Tips

1. Remember to protect your skin from the sun by applying a broad-spectrum sunscreen with at least SPF 30 daily.
2. Avoid heavy or oil-based skincare products, as they can further exacerbate oiliness in the T-zone.
3. Maintain a balanced diet and drink plenty of water to promote overall skin health.
4. Practise stress-reducing activities such as yoga or meditation, as stress can affect your skin's balance.

I hope it's now easier for you to recognise your skin type and take the necessary steps to nourish it accordingly, making your skin look plumper, shinier, and healthier.

3

The Skin Life Cycle

In my practice of over four decades, I have consulted and treated people of all ages. As we age, our skin undergoes various changes that are important to recognise and accept. In this chapter, we will explore the skin conditions commonly experienced by women in four different age groups. It can help us gain insight into the clear and noticeable differences that tell the story of ageing.

Here is an overview of some common changes that occur at different ages.

Adolescence: The skin is affected by hormonal changes, which lead to excess production of sebum, causing oiliness and acne. The skin is otherwise supple and firm.

20 to 35 years: During this age, women's endocrine system is at its peak, resulting in the over-activity of the sweat and oil glands, which causes excessive perspiration and oiliness. During this time many women experience enlarged pores and acne. In fact, some women experience the first signs of wrinkles during this time.

35 to 50 years: The skin glands become sluggish, leading to a thinner, less supple, and dry skin. Collagen production decreases, which can lead to sagging skin. As the skin's natural exfoliation system slows down, it can result in uneven and dull skin. Pigmentation can also be spotted on the skin. Additionally, broken capillaries and veins become noticeable.

50 years and above: The skin continues to lose collagen, resulting in further wrinkles and creases. During this time, the skin becomes extremely dry, and dark brown spots appear in several places. Age spots and other forms of pigmentation become more pronounced.

Ageing Gracefully: Skincare across the Ages

1 to 12 Years

If your child has normal skin without any dry spots or blackheads, there is no problem. But you would be wrong to think that your child's skin is fine and there is no need to take care of it. Always use a mild face wash with, preferably, soft water both in the day and at night. Apply a light moisturising baby lotion to protect the skin and keep it soft.

For soft water, boil some water and a little boric acid to it. Mix this solution with the water you want to soften.

Furthermore, we have known for a while now that exposure to ultraviolet radiation from the sun is cumulative, meaning that every ray of sunlight you get, whether at age one or fifty, adds up over time. However, it's only recently that we have discovered that an hour of sun exposure is far more damaging to a child's skin than to an adult's. Although your skin can recover to some extent if you avoid sun exposure for a few years, any damage caused by exposure can never be completely reversed. Thus, we should teach our children to use sunscreens from an early age to help protect their skin from harmful UV rays.

DIY Recipe: To make your sunscreen at home for your child, take both calamine and baby lotion in equal proportions. Add a pinch of zinc oxide to the mixture. Apply the lotion before your child steps outside.

To avoid sunburn, mix vinegar with olive oil in equal quantities and apply to the exposed areas. Leave it on for an hour before rinsing it off. Follow this process an hour before your child steps outside during the day.

Adolescence

During this time, the skin needs thorough because of the hormonal changes that take place in one's body. Puberty often leads to oily skin, resulting in blackheads, whiteheads, and acne. This is a result of the overactivity of the sebaceous glands.

To fight against the excess production of sebum, you can take some precautions.

Wash your face with warm water with a pH-balanced face wash. Nothing can make your skin better than washing it twice a day. After cleansing, spray some soda water on your face, or you can go for a non-alcoholic toner available in the market. Natural toners like cucumber or apple juice also work wonders.

In the morning, after cleansing your face with a mild face wash, freshen up your skin with rose water. Then apply a gel-based moisturiser or calamine lotion.

At night, remove your make-up with an oil-based make-up remover, cleanse, and use a toner.

DIY Recipe: You can use a face pack consisting of 1 beaten egg white mixed with a few drops of lemon juice. Keep it on for 15 minutes and then wash it off with lukewarm water. Apply this once in a week for best results.

Another change that the fluctuation in hormonal levels leads to in teenagers is acne. Due to the increased sebum production, pores get clogged, resulting in their inflammation.

Some of the precautions to be taken:

- Avoid products that contain petroleum jelly
- Choose a mild, pH-balanced face wash
- Avoid foods that are high in spicy or starch

Furthermore, follow a morning and nighttime skincare routine diligently. In the morning, after cleansing your face, apply a medicated anti-acne lotion, and let it dry naturally. Then move on to apply an anti-acne gel.

At night, make sure to remove your make-up or sunscreen and follow it up with a mild face wash. Then apply an overnight anti-acne gel.

20 to 35 Years

This is the time when your hormones are at their peak, resulting in the overactivity of both the oil and sweat glands. In fact, even your sense of smell and taste are at their most acute, and you are at your sexual peak.

Due to the overactivity of the sebaceous glands, extremely oily skin is one of the major skin concerns for many young women during their twenties and thirties. Another concern is the appearance of enlarged pores.

To control enlarged pores, apply a mixture of tomato juice and honey daily for ten minutes and then wash it off.

Furthermore, you must be extremely careful about the sun exposure. Always make sure to generously apply sunscreens and sunblock with an SPF of 30 or higher. This will help avoid the appearance of sunspots.

Lastly, fine lines also start appearing during this time. Keep your face well moisturised and hydrated, especially around the eyes and lips.

For under Eye Woes

If you are someone who has pigmentation around the eyes, there's an excellent but simple remedy. Take a thick slice of potato, make small holes all over it with a fork, and place it around your eyes. Alternatively, soak some cotton in warm tea and place it around the eyes.

For your eyelids, apply a drop of castor oil, as it helps keep the area supple and smooth. It also helps grow your eyelashes and eyebrows.

If you are also noticing signs of crow's feet, soak some breadcrumbs in milk and add a few drops of sweet almond oil. Wrap this mixture in a muslin cloth, close your eyes, and gently place it over your closed eyes.

35 to 50 Years

During this time, your skin gets thinner and loses its elasticity. It is also beginning to show changes in pigment as the complexion turns uneven and duller. You might also notice set groves around the upper lip, eyes, and forehead. Due to lack of collagen, your skin also sags, making you feel like you're wearing skin that is several sizes too big for you.

While you cannot avoid these changes, you can take appropriate care of your skin by sticking to a regular CTM routine, regularly massaging your face to keep the muscles and skin toned, and applying face packs to keep the skin hydrated. Additionally, regular facials will also help provide your face with much-needed nourishment. Make sure to use serums with hyaluronic acid and face oils to keep your skin moisturised.

DIY Recipe: To make your face oil, take 1 teaspoon of jojoba oil and add 2 drops of patchouli oil. Apply this regularly.

50 and Beyond

Our skin changes as we grow older. The skin exfoliates itself every three to four weeks until the twenties. However, in the mid-thirties and forties, this renewal process takes twice the time. In the fifties, it further slows down, leading to changes in the complexion like unevenness and dullness. In general, the vitality of the skin largely diminishes.

There is also a substantial decline in the number of blood vessels in the skin, resulting in the slowing down of circulation. The skin, therefore, becomes increasingly sensitive to both heat and cold. Although these changes are not evident to us daily, they do occur every day as we age.

Dry skin is also another major concern. When our skin starts to get seriously dry, we usually try to solve the problem by using a standard moisturiser. What we don't realise is that the process of cell replacement and natural lubricant production reduces as well. The key is to get the hydration back to how it used to be. Exfoliation is something that can greatly help, as it helps get rid of the dead skin cells, boosting cell division, and making skin cells perform more actively.

DIY Recipe 1: Take a pinch of alum, and some mashed

banana, and add a few drops of lavender oil and 1 teaspoon of whipped cream to it. Apply it on your face and neck and keep it on for about 20 minutes before washing it off with lukewarm water.

DIY Recipe 2: To boost cell division, tap your skin and use an almond scrub. Take a substantial pinch of powdered almonds and add 1/4 teaspoon of a cleansing cream of your choice. Mix it well and gently massage it into the skin. Wash it off once you're done.

DIY Recipe 3: You can also use a mix of finely powdered sugar and coconut oil to lightly massage your skin.

DIY Recipe 4: To make a nourishing mask, separate the egg yolk from the white. Beat the yolk with a little olive oil and add a drop of frankincense. Spread the mixture evenly all over your face and neck. Leave it on for 15 minutes and remove it with lukewarm water. Note: never use warm water as it would set the yolk.

DIY Recipe 5: To maintain the rhythm of cellular reproduction, apply a mixture of almond oil with a few drops of patchouli essential oil both morning and night. You can then follow it up with a moisturiser.

Ageing is natural, but we can choose to age gracefully while taking the utmost care of our skin and using products that provide ample hydration and nourishment.

4
Your Journey to Glowing Skin

When discussing skin conditions, we often consider complexion and texture. Complexion refers to the visual assessment of the skin's colour, tone, and clarity. Skin texture, on the other hand, describes how the skin feels to the touch. Together, complexion and texture reflect the overall character and health of the skin.

Factors Affecting Skin Complexion and Texture

As explained in the previous chapter, different skin types have different complexion and texture. Genetics and age also play a crucial role in determining one's skin characteristics, resulting in unique differences for everyone.

Furthermore, extreme weather conditions, improper skincare, the use of unsuitable cosmetics, and certain skin issues such as acne and pigmentation can impact the skin's colour, tone, and texture, possibly leading to adverse effects.

What Makes My Skin Dull and Lifeless?

One of the most common skin issues people face is the appearance of dullness and uneven skin tone. This usually happens due to the over-absorption of melanin by the topmost cell layer of our skin. Melanin is produced in the basal cell layer, and dead cells on the surface absorb this pigment.

A noticeable deterioration in skin is observed with age. Reduced blood circulation, decreased activity of oil and sweat glands, and degeneration of body tissues lead to dryness and wrinkles on the skin. This decline in skin rejuvenation and improper shedding of the dead cells also affect one's complexion and texture.

The aspects of skin complexion and texture that require our utmost attention include skin colour, clarity, and issues such as excessive dryness, roughness, and oiliness. There are a host of potent home-made recipes that can improve our complexion and enhance the texture of our skin.

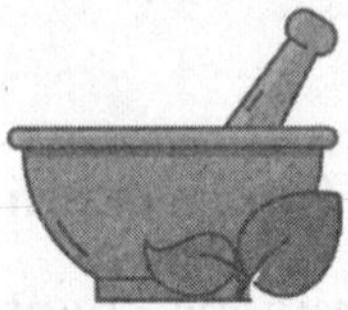

DIY Recipes for Radiant Skin

Recipe 1: Instead of using soap, use gram flour (equal quantities of green gram and Bengal gram) mixed in milk or rice water. Gently scrub it on your face (and body) and rinse it with clear water. This is an excellent recipe to clear the skin. Use this cleanser at least once or twice a week.

Recipe 2: Mix a pinch of turmeric, 1 tablespoon of milk powder, and half a lemon juice in two tablespoons of honey to make a paste. Apply it on your face and leave it on till it dries.

Recipe 3: Take equal quantities of black and white cumin seeds and make a thick paste with cream of the milk. Apply this paste all over your face and wash it off after 20 minutes. Use this mask at least twice a week for maximum effect.

Recipe 4: To remove dead skin, take 1/2 cup of seedless grapes, add 1 teaspoon of lemon juice, and 1 tablespoon of milk powder. Mix this with rose water. Apply it on your face and wash it off after 15 to 20 minutes.

Recipe 5: Take a sweet lime and cut it into two. Now, rub one half on the face gently. Squeeze the other half in a cup of water, add a little rock salt, and drink it. Do it regularly for six to eight weeks to observe a remarkable improvement.

Recipe 6: To get rid of blackheads and acne blemishes, make a fine paste of turmeric root and mustard seeds and apply it on the affected areas each night. You will notice the blackheads and whiteheads gradually fade away.

DIY Recipes for Improved Texture

To improve your skin texture if you have oily skin, follow these easy, home-made recipes:

Recipe 1: Use an oatmeal and sandalwood scrub (1 teaspoon oatmeal and ¼ teaspoon sandalwood powder) to cleanse the skin.

Recipe 2: Apply the mixture of 1/4 teaspoon vinegar in a glass of water to tone your skin.

Recipe 3: Cut some slices of raw potatoes, place them all over the face, and leave them on for 15 minutes. Use the recipe regularly for a smooth and moist texture.

To moisturise your dry and flaky skin, along with improving its texture, follow these DIY tips:

Recipe 1: After cleansing the skin with a cleanser, tone it with rose water.

Recipe 2: Apply half a teaspoon of glycerine to which a few drops of vitamin E oil or almond oil have been added. Rinse off after 20 minutes. Use this moisturising preparation on the face for a soft and moist look.

Recipe 3: Warm a teaspoon of honey and mix in a squeeze of lemon. Apply this all over your face and neck and wash it off after 20 minutes. Use this mask once a week for smooth and soft skin texture.

Some Beneficial Tips

- Yoghurt is an ideal ingredient to massage skin with, as it can soothe both dry and oily skin.
- Drinking a glass of water mixed with lime juice can improve the skin's texture and brighten it.
- Regularly consuming white radish and carrot juice can increase your vitamin A levels, which is significant for a smooth texture.
- Honey contains vitamin B-complex, which is important for healthy skin texture and colour.
- A diet of cucumber, onion, and fenugreek improves the complexion, making it brighter.

Things to Remember

To prevent damage to your skin barrier, you should avoid:

- Poor quality lipstick and blushers with stainers
- Creams that are highly alkaline
- Bleaching and lightening creams containing mercury
- Cleansing with strong soaps
- Popping pustules and picking on your acne

5
Understanding Common Skin Concerns

In this chapter, I will be discussing the most common skin concerns that people face at some point in their lives. Dealing with skin woes can be mentally and emotionally draining. However, understanding these issues and the different ways to address them can make the journey easier.

Most individuals experience some form of skin issues, regardless of age. For teenagers, it could be acne and open pores, while older individuals may experience pigmentation, under-eye problems, and rapid ageing of the skin. Read on to find some solid solutions to your skin issues.

Acne

Acne is the most common skin disorder, which predictably occurs first during the teenage years. Research states that a recognisable form of acne affects over 70 per cent of adolescents. Blackheads and whiteheads are closely associated with the hyperactivity of the oil glands, leading to congested pores. Seborrhoea or excessive oiliness on the skin's surface is the general precondition to the formation of acne.

It occurs when the male hormone, testosterone, in the body becomes overtly dominant during puberty. This activity of the oil glands, which is controlled and regulated by male hormones, fervently increases. To cope with the overproduction of oil secretions, the skin must manage the disposal of waste. As the flow of oil increases, the pores enlarge, leading to open pores.

How to Identify Acne?

Acne can be identified by checking the following skin conditions:

- Excessive oiliness
- Whiteheads, which sometimes appear to be inflamed
- Blackheads
- Enlarged pores
- Little bumps under the skin—mostly in clusters

Where Does Acne Appear?

Acne mostly affects the face, back, chest, and shoulders. This is because these parts of the body have a high concentration of oil glands and hair follicles, which can lead to the development of acne. If left untreated, acne can spread all over your body and turn into a severe infection.

Types of Acne

Acne comes in diverse forms, and recognising the types can help in identifying and treating the condition effectively. Below are some common types of acne.

Mild Acne

This is the most common type of acne, which greatly affects teenagers. This type of acne does not persist for long without breaks. It may last a few months, disappear for some weeks, and then reappear.

Mild acne conditions are the easiest to treat. It can potentially turn into a severe form, with the most likely reason being improper or inadequate skincare. Furthermore, scarring in mild acne is uncommon; few pits remain after the spots have dried up.

Moderate Acne (Acne Vulgaris)

When many papules develop in the late teens and early twenties, the prevalence of whiteheads also increases. In about 10 per cent of cases, individuals with mild acne notice their condition worsening due to the prolonged presence of acne and severe oily skin, leading to moderate acne. The affected spots turn red due to ruptured blood vessels. Generally, this type of acne improves with minimal scarring.

Severe Acne (Chronic)

In this case, red acne spots are higher in number and larger in size. They are not only infected but painful to touch, especially when compared to moderate acne. Only a small proportion of individuals suffer from severe or chronic acne.

Here, the entire face, shoulders, and back can be affected. It typically takes a long time to treat this condition, with a high chance of scarring if the acne is picked.

Picker's Acne

Some young women develop spots that are quite unnoticeable to the naked eye. Upon close examination, they may look different from the typical acne. However, the central part of the acne is not like its tip but is covered by a scab instead.

This occurs because the spot has been frequently picked and scratched.

Cosmetics and Fringe Acne

This occurs mainly on the forehead and is mostly due to the presence of excessive oil and grease on the skin's surface, which, in turn, clogs the hair follicles.

Factors Aggravating Acne

Several factors can exacerbate acne, such as:

- Prolonged stress and anxiety
- Vitamin B12 deficiency
- Hormonal changes
- Poor skincare habits
- Continual touch and picking
- Excessive consumption of fried foods
- Change in weather
- Iodine-rich foods
- Hysterectomy and menopause
- Genetics

Managing Acne

There are two broad aspects of treating acne:

Medical Treatment

Medical treatment is suggested only in cases of chronic or severe acne. All advice should only be taken from a dermatologist, who will prescribe drugs that can applied to the affected areas or consumed orally. These medications will largely focus on:

- Cutting down the bacteria in hair follicles and the skin's surface
- Opening the hair follicles by removing blackheads
- Reducing acne inflammation

Daily Skincare

I cannot emphasise the importance of following a daily skincare routine enough. One must not skip any of the steps.

Morning and Night care

- Wash your hands thoroughly
- Wash your face with a medicated or antiseptic cleanser
- Spray or dab your face with a non-alcoholic toner, which will help freshen up your skin and reduce excess oil
- Apply a medicated gel on the affected areas to dry and heal the acne
- Apply a calamine lotion mixed with a drop of clove and mint oil on the affected areas

Mid-day

- Spray your face with a non-alcoholic toner
- Reapply the medicated gel on blemishes

Twice Weekly

- To control blackheads and avoid clogging the pores,

deeply cleanse your face with a medicated face wash. Massage gently for a few seconds and rinse thoroughly.

Dos and Don'ts

- Do not rub, squeeze, or pick at pustules
- Avoid using oil-based creams, ointments, and make-up products
- Religiously follow the skincare routine
- Try to live your life as stress-free as possible
- Supplement your diet with additional vitamin B12
- Avoid deep-fried food
- In case of severe acne, consult a doctor

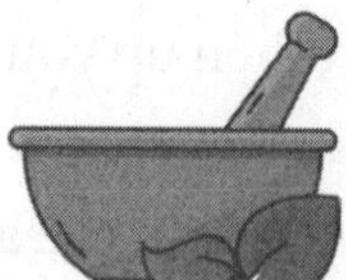

DIY Remedies for Managing and Soothing Acne

Cleanser

Recipe 1: Dissolve 1 teaspoon of Epsom salts (Magnesium Sulphate) in a cup of hot water. Apply this to the affected areas with a cotton pad.

Recipe 2: A papaya-mint tea bag dissolved in a cup of hot water and applied on the acne also acts as a desincrusting lotion.

Toner

Recipe 1: Add about 2–3 drops of tea tree oil to a mug of cold water. Rinse your face with this antibacterial concoction.

Pack

Recipe 1: Add 2 pods of crushed garlic and 1 teaspoon of calamine to 2 teaspoons of egg white. Mix in 2 drops of tea tree oil and 1 drop of Patchouli to this mixture. Apply this on your face and leave it on your face for 20 minutes.

Moisturiser

Recipe 1: Mix 1/4 teaspoon of vinegar, 5 drops of glycerine, and 2 drops of tea tree oil into a bottle of rose water. Use this to keep your skin hydrated.

To Dry Acne

Recipe 1: Dab some tea tree oil on the affected areas and regularly apply it until the acne dries up. It may initially sting, but it will stop the infection from spreading further.

To Lighten Scars

Recipe 1: Take a bunch of freshly washed green grapes. Sprinkle 1 tablespoon of alum and 1 teaspoon of salt. Wrap the grapes in foil and bake in the oven on the slow mode for 15 minutes. Squeeze out the grape juice and apply it to your face. Rinse off after 15 minutes with lukewarm water.

Recipe 2: After cleansing your face, mix 1 teaspoon of water with a drop of patchouli oil. Apply this mixture to the acne scars.

Myths and Facts

Myth: Improper hygiene is a leading cause of acne

It is both true and false. If proper cleansing is not carried out, it can aggravate the acne. However, if the appropriate hygiene routine is followed but with the use of harsh or excessive cleansing and scrubbing, it can ironically worsen the condition.

Myth: Long hair can aggravate acne

It is not the length but the improper hair cleansing that can worsen the acne.

Myth: Girls are more prone to acne than boys

False! In fact, it is the other way around. Acne is more common in boys because of the dominance of male hormones like testosterone.

Myth: Acne is contagious

No. The trouble-making bacteria are buried deep within the skin.

Myth: Masturbation makes acne worse

This is false and is groundless.

Myth: Eating certain foods can cause or aggravate acne

This is partially true. Research shows that traditionally forbidden foods like fried foods, chocolates, colas, and dairy products do not adversely affect the presence or aggravation of acne. However, foods rich in iodide, such as cabbage, spinach, and wheat germ can trigger acne-like eruptions.

Open Pores

Our skin has thousands of tiny openings, known as pores, that are not visible to the naked eye. These pores carry out the important functions of eliminating water, salts, and uric acid and secreting oil from our bodies.

The problem of enlarged pores is commonly associated with excessive oiliness and the presence of acne. The excessive oiliness of the skin is, in turn, triggered by hormonal changes in the body.

Causes behind Enlarged Pores

Three main factors are directly responsible for the formation of enlarged pores:

1. Deliberate Picking and Touching of Acne: Constantly touching the acne results in scars and pits. Artificial openings created in the skin to release effusion from whitehead pustules by squeezing can turn into pits and uneven indentations.
2. Improper Cleansing: Proper cleansing is crucial in every skincare routine. If not removed properly, dead skin cells, make-up, and grease can accumulate in the skin pores, restraining oil flow. These oil deposits, in turn, can attract grime and grease, applying pressure on the pores and widening them.
3. Use of Wrong Products: Beauty soaps enriched with oil, oil-based make-up products, and creams worsen oily skin conditions and are, therefore, not recommended. Such cosmetics can aggravate acne and lead to enlarged skin pores.

Treatment of Enlarged Pores

While you cannot permanently change their size, you can minimise their appearance with some strategies, such as proper cleansing and frequent toning of the skin. Many vegetables, fruits, and herbs also help reduce the appearance of enlarged pores.

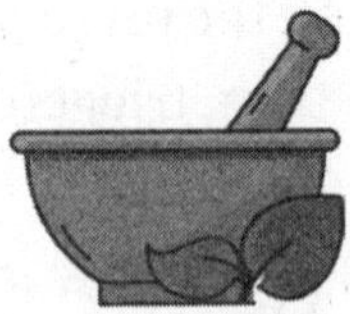

DIY Remedies for Managing Enlarged Pores

Recipe 1: Peel 1 cucumber and whip it up with 2 egg whites. Add 1 teaspoon of lemon juice, 2 tablespoons of brandy, and 1/2 teaspoon of ground mint (optional). In case the mixture is watery, add some Kaolin (white clay) to make it thick. Apply a generous application of the paste on the areas with large pores and leave it on for 20 minutes. Rinse off with clear water. Use this recipe at least twice a week.

Recipe 2: To 1 tablespoon of Kaolin, add a pinch of camphor, 1 tablespoon of honey, and a few drops of brandy. Apply it on the face and leave it on for 20 minutes before rinsing it off. If you don't have camphor, alum (*phitkari*) powder works equally well. Use the recipe daily.

Recipe 3: Make a thick paste of oatmeal in some buttermilk or cucumber juice. Apply it on the face for 15 minutes and rinse it off. Apart from treating the large pores, this mask also helps in improving the texture of the skin.

Dos and Don'ts

- Apply minimum make-up if your skin is extremely oily
- Cleanse your face at least three times a day with a mild soap and water
- Use water-based cosmetics and powder-based make-up products
- Religiously follow home-made cosmetic care
- Do not pick or squeeze acne, whiteheads, pustules, or papules as it will only make them worse

The home care toning routine is a convenient way of dealing with large pores. It is important to utilise the astringent qualities of these recipes to shrink the pores.

Apart from the aforementioned home-made recipes, vinegar in water, milk, yoghurt, tomato, and almond are some of the other food products that can effectively minimise the appearance of enlarged pores. They can be used in the form of lotions or face masks.

PIGMENTATION

Women, in their 40s, typically approach me, distraught over pigmentation. They seek immediate solutions, but I always advise them to have patience. The issue of pigmentation arises from excessive production of melanin and darkening of the skin or a loss of colour and pigment—either across the entire body or in patches.

The reason pigmentation is more prevalent amongst women in their 40s is related to the endocrinal changes that occur during this age. The severity of pigmentation is linked to several diseases and disorders.

What Causes Excessive Pigmentation?

The hormones produced by our endocrinal system influence the production of the colouring agent, melanin, in our skin. Certain internal conditions, such as menopause, and internal disorders have adverse effects on the endocrinal system, leading to hormonal imbalance, which results in the excessive secretion of melanin.

Additionally, excessive keratinisation, a condition characterised by the presence of dead cells (not exfoliated), on the skin's surface leads to the darkening of complexion. Our scaly skin surface absorbs excessive melanin, therefore, appearing dark.

In cases of liver disorder, it is found that excess bilirubin seeps out of the blood vessels into the spaces between the tissue cells. This imparts a yellow complexion to the skin.

Internal Disorders that Cause Pigmentation

To understand the unusual occurrence of pigmentation, we need to first understand these internal disorders:

a. Pigmentation of the skin is a symptom common to several internal disorders. We need to correctly diagnose the diseases and disorders to effectively clear up the pigmentation.

b. A bronze pigmentation appears across the body due to the over-absorption of iron from the food in the intestinal tract.

c. The skin can gain a brownish pigmentation as well as the colours of other compounds that are malabsorbed. For instance, women using nasal drops regularly absorb excess quantities of silver present in them and can develop a silver-grey pigmentation in the skin.
d. Jaundice is another cause, wherein the skin turns yellow due to the presence of excess bile in the blood and body tissue.
e. Seldom, during pregnancy, dark brown spots appear on the face. This occurs due to the hormonal imbalances caused during the pregnancy.
f. The skin can turn bluish or purplish due to the lack of oxygen in the blood. Women suffering from pneumonia, chronic diseases, and other heart problems notice this type of pigmentation.
g. Menopause leads to a decline in hormonal levels, which, in turn, affects the secretion of melanin. In the case of surgical menopause—by removing the ovaries or the uterus—this pigmentation can be more obvious and severe.
h. Amoebiasis is a chronic intestinal disorder that can cause excessive purging of the bowels, leading to dehydration and a pale complexion.
i. Deficiencies in iron, calcium, vitamin A, E, and B Complex can result in patchy and spotty discolouration of the skin.

External Factors that Cause Pigmentation

Three major external factors can cause pigmentation of the skin:

a. Excessive Sun: Overexposure to the sun without protection can lead to the tanning of the skin, resulting in a darker skin tone. The ultraviolet rays penetrate the skin, damaging its cells.
b. Use of Wrong Cosmetics: Certain make-up products containing chemical colours or creams with mercury can adversely affect the skin's surface. This, in turn, can cause pigmentation.
c. Oral Medications: Drugs prescribed for high blood pressure, asthma, diabetes, insomnia, birth control, and acne can unfavourably impact the skin. Often, these drugs can cause pigmentation spots to appear on the skin.

Clearing up Pigmentation

There is no magical or instant solution to treat pigmentation. The treatment process depends on how old and acute the pigmentation is. Bleaching and skin peeling are the two most effective methods followed by cosmetologists to resolve excessive pigmentation. The good thing about these methods is that they can be done at home, safely and easily, with niacinamide and zinc.

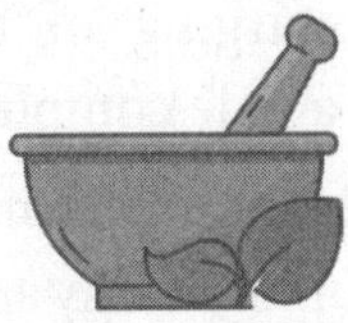

DIY Recipes for Managing Pigmentation

Bleach

Milk is one of the most natural and effective bleaching co-agents. Powdered milk works best.

Recipe 1: Take 2 tablespoons of milk powder, some papaya pulp, and a squeeze of lemon to make a paste.

Add a few drops of glycerine to this paste and apply it to the dark spots. Leave it on for about 20 minutes and then rinse it off.

If your skin feels dry after rinsing, use a generous amount of moisturising lotion.

Recipe 2: Both niacinamide and zinc are effective in lightening the blemishes and highly pigmented spots. Regularly apply a mixture of zinc oxide and aloe vera gel on the spots.

Recipe 3: Break vitamin E capsules and add in a few drops of castor oil. Apply it on the deeply pigmented areas.

Scrubs and Masks for Skin Peeling

Recipe 1: Mix 1/2 teaspoon of plain sugar granules in your cleanser and gently work it into the skin. Make sure to especially concentrate on the affected spots. Once the sugar is absorbed into the skin, rinse your face with hot water, then with warm water, and finally with cold water. If you have oily skin, use the scrub twice a week. For dry skin, use it once a week.

Recipe 2: Crush some almonds or oats and apply the granular paste on the face for a few minutes. Rinse off with cool water.

Recipe 3: Grate some papaya skin and mix 1/2 cup of Multani mitti and the oil of 2 vitamin A capsules. Apply this paste on your face and rinse off after 20 minutes.

Recipe 4: Take some carrot pulp and mix some Multani mitti to make a thick paste. Crush a vitamin C tablet and add it to the paste. Apply this mixture and leave it on for 20 minutes before washing it off. You can use this at least once a week.

Note: Ensure that your skin doesn't get too dry from these treatments. Moisturise well after using these treatments. Buttermilk is a gentle bleach.

Dos and Don'ts

- If you experience uneven skin tone in patches, consider adding iron and calcium to your diet under the guidance of a doctor.
- If your complexion is pale and dull, add vitamin A to your diet to improve colour
- In case of severe, long-lasting pigmentation, consult a physician
- Have a vitamin B-complex capsule daily. It is water-soluble, which makes it harmless as the excess is easily flushed out of the body
- Avoid using cosmetics with colouring agents as they can darken the skin
- Use minimal make-up
- Apply a sunblock cream before stepping out in the sun
- Avoid using oral birth control pills and sleeping pills. For asthma and diabetes, use only the prescribed dose
- Avoid distress and anxiety as much as possible

UNDER-EYE ISSUES

Most of us have experienced under-eye issues, such as dark circles and fine lines, at some point in our lives. Factors such as lack of sleep, various illnesses, stress, and excessive screen time, contribute to under-eye problems.

The delicate skin surrounding the eyes is approximately ten times thinner than the rest of your face. Over time, the skin's elasticity diminishes, and the thinness intensifies due to the gradual decline in collagen production. Additional factors like exposure to the sun without protection, smoking, and environmental elements can worsen these effects. The eye contour experiences continuous motion, with blinking alone accounting for around 10,000 movements each day. Furthermore, various facial expressions like smiling and squinting can impact the eye area, resulting in fine lines or crow's feet. Let's explore the various under-eye issues and ways to combat them.

Dark Circles

This area may appear as shades of blue, purple, brown, or black, depending on your natural skin colour. Dark circles under your eyes may make you appear exhausted or older than you are.

The likely causes of dark circles are:

- Genetics
- Dermatitis
- Rubbing your eyes
- Lack of sleep

- Hyperpigmentation
- Dehydration
- Lifestyle factors

Managing Dark Circles

You can compress the area with cold, green tea bags on the eyes for about 15 minutes. Additionally, getting enough sleep, at least 8 hours, is extremely important. Make sure to take breaks and rest your eyes completely, especially if your work requires excessive screen time, for quick under-eye skin rejuvenation.

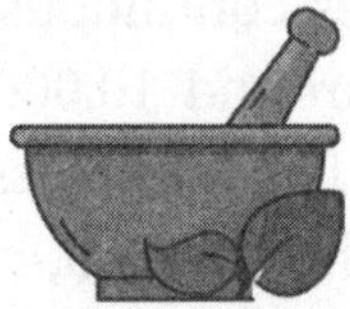

DIY Recipes for Dealing with Dark Circles

Recipe 1: Place either grated potato or cucumber slices on the eyes for 15 minutes. Alternatively, you can squeeze out their juice, dip cotton pads in it, and place the damp cotton pads on the eyes.

Recipe 2: Take some cold milk, preferably raw, soak cotton pads in it, and place them on the eyes. Repeat this process for 15–20 minutes.

Recipe 3: Take some freshly extracted aloe vera gel, massage it around the eyes for 2–3 minutes and leave it for 10–15 minutes. Rinse off with regular water.

Crow's Feet

As mentioned earlier, the skin beneath your eyes is exceptionally thin and delicate. With age, the natural decline in collagen production causes the skin to lose its firmness. Unfortunately, this process is particularly noticeable around the eye area, resulting in lines at the outer corners of your eyes. These are referred to as lateral canthal lines, commonly known as crow's feet or laugh lines. These delicate lines and wrinkles develop when the small muscles around the outer edges of your eyes contract while experiencing a range of emotions that affect your facial expressions, including laughter, stress, grief, and sadness.

Likely causes of crow's feet:

- Ageing
- Exposure to UV rays
- Smoking
- Dehydration of the skin
- Medication
- Improper skincare routine
- Less protein and fat intake
- Repetitive facial expressions
- Genetics

Managing Crow's Feet

Using moisturisers, eye creams, and eye gels specifically designed to target wrinkles and promote skin hydration can help improve the appearance of crow's feet over time. Look for products containing ingredients like retinol, peptides, hyaluronic acid, and antioxidants.

Keep the skin around your eyes well-hydrated and moisturised. Do not skip SPF when stepping out in the sun. Also, ensure a moderate consumption of alcohol and avoid smoking.

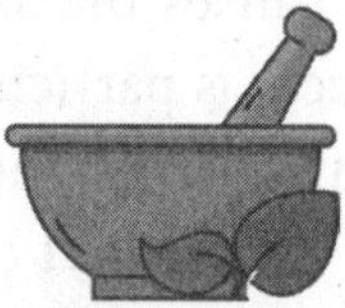

DIY Recipes for Managing Crow's Feet

Recipe 1: Mix 1 teaspoon of almond oil and 1 teaspoon of castor oil. Gently massage this oil mix around your eyes for 10–15 minutes.

Recipe 2: Add some breadcrumbs to some milk and create a thick paste. Take two cotton pads, spread the mixture between the pads, and place them on the eyes for 20 minutes. Also, apply a little almond oil around the eyes before placing the pads.

Recipe 3: Take 1 teaspoon of coffee and 1 teaspoon of honey or aloe vera gel (if you're allergic to honey). Mix well apply it around the eyes and leave it on for 10–15 minutes. Rinse off with regular water.

Recipe 4: Take 1 teaspoon of olive oil and gently massage the skin around your eyes with your ring fingers for about 10 minutes.

Puffy or Baggy Eyes

Under-eye bags develop when the supportive tissues and muscles that hold your eyelids weaken over time. This weakening can cause the skin to sag, allowing the fat that normally surrounds the eyes to shift downwards. Additionally, the area beneath your eyes can accumulate fluid, resulting in a puffy or swollen appearance.

Likely causes of puffy or baggy eyes:

- Ageing
- Fluid retention, especially upon waking or after a salty meal
- Lack of sleep
- Allergies
- Smoking
- Genetics—under-eye bags can run in families
- Medical conditions

Taking Care

Quit or reduce smoking and alcohol consumption as much as possible. Add green tea, detox water, juices, soups, etc., to your diet. Additionally, control your salt consumption before going to bed as this leads to puffiness around the eyes.

Consume foods that are rich in collagen by increasing your protein intake. Furthermore, use eye products that can aid in increasing the production of collagen.

Make sure to regularly compress the area around your eyes—use a cold compress, hot compress, or a combination of both. For a cold compress, start by placing two tea bags in a cup of hot water and allow them to steep for 3–5 minutes. Afterwards, remove the tea bags from the cup and let them cool down in the refrigerator for approximately 20 minutes. Once chilled, apply the tea bags to the under-eye area and leave them for about 15 minutes.

To create a hot compress, soak two tea bags in warm water, then gently squeeze out the excess water. Place the warm tea bags on your eyes and repeat this process for 15 minutes.

If desired, you can combine the hot and cold compress methods. Prepare two cold tea bags and two warm tea bags. Begin by placing the warm tea bags on the eyes for 2–3 minutes, then switch to the cold tea bags for another 2–3 minutes. Repeat this process three times.

It is crucial to grasp and tackle common skincare worries to keep your skin healthy and glowing. Recognising issues like acne, dryness, sensitivity, and signs of ageing allows you to customise your skincare regimen to deal with these challenges effectively. Adopting a holistic strategy involving thorough cleansing, hydration, protection, and specific treatments can ease these concerns and boost skin health and self-assurance. Keep in mind that consistency and patience are important, as skincare is a process towards achieving your desired outcomes.

6

Skin Defence for Every Season

The skin changes according to seasons, and this applies to all skin types. In fact, there is never a time of the year when you can relax with your beauty regime. You go through all the trouble in summer to make sure that your skin and hair are thoroughly protected against the sun and heat only to discover that on the return of the colder months, your skin is dry, parched and lacks moisture and you are back where you started. Skincare varies with seasons for all skin types.

In this chapter, we will explore how the change in the weather affects your skin and ways you can protect it from the various changes. Here's a guide to skin defence for every season.

Winter

Winter brings forth its own set of problems. As the air gets cooler, glands just below the surface of the skin become relatively inactive, resulting in dryness. Furthermore, cold winds lead to dry red patches along with tight, flaky skin.

Even inside your warm and cosy home, you could be doing your skin more harm than good by sitting too close to the heater, as the dry air drains your skin of its natural moisture. This can further lead to flaky, red skin along with chapped lips.

How to Protect Your Skin in Winter?

The best way to tackle dryness is to completely cease using soap. Most of the soaps are extremely drying and using them would only add to your woes. Instead, opt for a gentle cleansing lotion or cleansing cream as these would help moisturise your skin. However, if you are a dedicated soap lover, then go for a mild soap with a moisturising base, such as glycerine.

If you must use a heater, keep a pot of water over your heater to keep the air in your home moist. If possible, leave a window slightly open to allow some fresh air inside.

Moisturising is a crucial step in your winter skincare routine. During this time, the skin usually loses moisture more quickly than it can replenish it. Your skin must be protected with extra-hydrating creams, as they can help lock in the moisture below the skin's surface and act as a barrier against external conditions. It's essential to apply moisturisers twice a day—once in the morning and once before you go to bed—after cleansing and toning.

Additionally, use a heavy-duty moisturiser in winter, and apply it while your skin is still damp. Make sure to gently massage it on your face in an upward and outward motion.

Make sure to wash your face at least half an hour before going out into the cold. Your skin loves water, but the water that has moisturised your face will crack the skin when it meets the cold air.

Your make-up base, too, plays a substantial role in protecting your face from the cold, especially if it is a hydrating foundation. They work in a similar manner as a moisturiser, albeit on a smaller scale. However, you have the added advantage of a foundation to even out your skin tone.

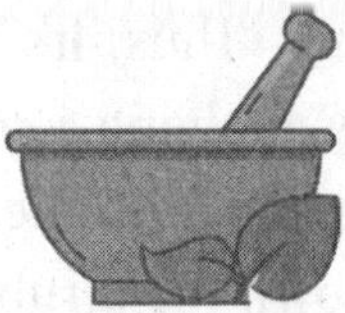

To camouflage unevenness and dark circles, use a concealer under your foundation for that smooth finish.

Home-Made Recipes for Winter

Recipe 1: Begin your routine with a good home-made cleanser, such as a mixture of cream of the milk and a pinch of turmeric powder.

Recipe 2: Every night, before going to bed, take 1 tablespoon of cream of milk and mix in a few drops of glycerine, castor oil, and rose water. Blend well and apply it all over your face, neck, and hands. Leave it overnight. Wash it off with cold water the next morning.

This home-made formula contains oil, which can combine with our natural oil to insulate and form a protective barrier on the skin surface, keeping moisture in and the harmful effects of the environment out.

Recipe 3: It's important to add a hydrating mask to your routine. Make one at home by taking 1/4 cup of yoghurt, 1 teaspoon of honey, 1 tablespoon of milk powder, and a small piece of mashed banana. Leave it on for 10 minutes, then wash it off with cold water. Do this once a week for the best results.

Tips for slick lips: As lips have no oil glands of their own, it makes them extremely prone to chapping and cracking, especially in cold weather. Thus, it's important to take extra care and protect them by applying a coat of Vaseline overnight and using a hydrating lip salve in the morning. The salve can be applied either on its own for a subtle sheen or underneath your lipstick.

However, if your lips are dry and chapped, avoid applying lipstick as it will dry them further. Also, apply a moisturiser on your lips several times a day to keep them hydrated and plump. You can then move on to applying lip gloss or a lip balm of your choice. Always seal your products with sunscreen.

DIY Recipe 1: Exfoliate your lips with a mix of butter and powdered sugar.

DIY Recipe 2: To make your lips soft, crush some rose petals and add a little butter. Apply this generously on your lips before going to bed.

Summer

Summer can be challenging for maintaining healthy skin due to various environmental factors. Depending on the region, the warm weather often brings about an increase in humidity or dryness. This can lead to a range of skin issues, like excess oil production, moisture depletion, sunburns, and dullness. These conditions can also contribute to the appearance of acne, open pores, and blackheads.

Moreover, the type of summer you experience plays a crucial role in determining the appropriate skincare routine. For instance, a hot and humid summer may lead to more oily skin, while a hot and dry summer could result in drier skin that requires extra hydration. Adapting your skincare regimen according to these conditions can help manage the impact of summer on your skin and maintain a healthy, glowing complexion.

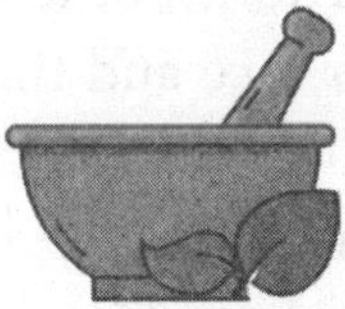

Home-Made Recipes to Protect Your Skin During Hot and Dry Summer

Recipe 1: Mash a ripe banana or a watermelon, mix in 1 teaspoon of milk powder and 1/4 teaspoon of honey. Apply the mixture to a clean face and neck and leave it on for 20 minutes before washing it off with cold water.

To combat the dry summer heat, make this moisturising pack and use it twice a week. This nourishing mask is good for dark skin that becomes grey and dull due to the heat and parching winds.

Recipe 2: In summer, even at your oiliest, do not excessively cleanse your face with harsh soaps. Instead, use strong astringents and abrasive pore-minimising grains. Try a pack with oatmeal and tomato juice to shrink the appearance of pores and exfoliate the dead skin cells.

Recipe 3: Take 1 tablespoon of tomato juice and mix enough oatmeal to make a thin paste. Add 1 drop of essential oil of peppermint oil. Apply to damp skin, while avoiding the eye and mouth areas.

Leave it on for 5–10 minutes before wiping it off with a damp cotton cloth or sponge. Then, move on to wash your face with cold water.

Recipe 4: To reduce unwanted grease from your face, add 1 teaspoon of table salt to a bottle filled with water. Spray this concoction on your face and then gently wipe it with a soft towel.

Additionally, rubbing slices of unpeeled cucumber or potato on the face can reduce shine.

Recipe 5: If you swim for hours at a stretch, apply a protective barrier of Vaseline. Add a few drops of lavender oil to it.

Exposure to chlorine can damage the skin and cause it to lose its moisture. When the skin is subjected to water for a prolonged period, the dead cells on the surface absorb moisture and shrink when they dry out. This can lead to dry and dehydrated skin. Using a protective product can help to prevent this and maintain the skin's natural moisture balance. Lavender oil also helps prevent burning.

When your skin is unprotected, it can burn within minutes of sun exposure. To protect your skin, you must use sunscreen that guards against UV rays. Alternatively, you could use a sunscreen that completely blocks the sun's rays.

If your skin is especially dry or sensitive dry or sensitive, look for products containing pure aminobenzoic acid and benzophenones, but avoid those with alcohol. Regardless of your skin type, sunscreens should always be applied over moisturiser and under make-up.

Spraying tea water on your face before applying moisturiser acts as a good home-made sunscreen for a short period when you are out in the sun.

No sunscreen should provide a false sense of security. Even the most potent products still allow some radiation to reach the skin. For complete protection, use a sunblock containing zinc oxide or titanium dioxide. These ingredients are opaque, which block and scatter light. Furthermore, they are often tinted to match skin tones for a more aesthetically pleasing look.

Recipe 6: For sunburns, add a few drops of lavender essential oil to iced water and apply to the affected areas. Iced milk and cucumber juice can also soothe the afflicted areas. Apply either of these mixtures every 2 to 4 hours.

Recipe 7: To remove tan and brighten dull skin, mix 1 tablespoon of powdered oatmeal with enough sour yoghurt to make a paste. Add some cucumber or grape juice to it. Massage this pack onto the tanned areas and leave it on for half an hour. Wash it off and follow it up with a moisturiser.

Recipe 8: Some individuals can notice a sudden appearance of freckles and skin discolouration during summer. Mix the powdered root of manjistha (India madder) with honey and apply it to the affected areas. This pack can considerably lighten the unevenness.

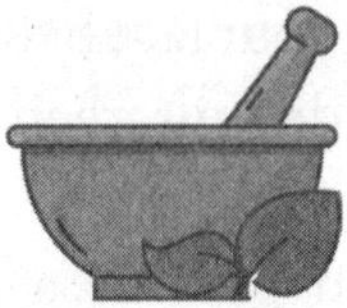

DIY Recipes to Protect Your Skin in Heat and Humidity

Recipe 1: Cleanse your skin often. Mix Multani mitti, channa ka atta (gram flour), and sandalwood powder in equal quantities. Store this mixture in an airtight container. To use, mix 1 teaspoon of this scrub with water to create a paste. Gently rub it on your skin. This helps rid the skin of flakes and dirt. Use this exfoliating scrub three times a week.

Use seasonal fruits as facial masks because they are economical and highly moisturising. Crush the pulp or blend the fruit and apply it as quickly as possible before the vitamins lose their potency. Grapes are rich in sugar, vitamins, and mineral salts. Apply them around the eyes and mouth to help moisturise, detoxify, and nourish the skin.

Recipe 2: Rubbing papaya on blackheads and uneven or sallow skin can be useful and brighten up the skin.

Recipe 3: Cucumber is cooling in nature and can improve a dull and greasy complexion. Apply a mix of cucumber juice with 1 teaspoon of rose water.

Recipe 4: Applying watermelon juice onto the face and neck instantly freshens up the skin.

Recipe 5: Gently tapping coconut water into the skin helps brighten the skin along with getting rid of any heat rash. Leave it on for about 15 minutes and wash it off with cool water.

Recipe 6: Make refreshing eye pads from thick slices of cucumber or cotton pads soaked in milk (iced). To relieve itchy, reddened eyes, use chilled raw potato slices. Place over eyelids and rest for 10 minutes.

Bathing Care

Recipe 1: Add a cup of buttermilk to your bath water to help minimise the appearance of pores.

Recipe 2: Mix 2 teaspoons of salt, 1 1/2 teaspoons of almond oil, and 1/2 teaspoon of malt vinegar. Apply this on your body before taking a bath. This bath formula will nourish and soothe your skin.

Recipe 3: To prevent tanning, take almond oil and malt vinegar in equal quantities and apply it to your body an hour before taking a shower/bath.

Recipe 3: To soothe sunburnt areas, use a head-to-toe yoghurt mask. Leave it on for 10 minutes and then take a shower with cold water. This will provide instant relief.

Recipe 4: Rubbing ice cubes wrapped in tissue on pulse points, such as wrists and ankles, can provide instant energy and boost your skin.

Recipe 5: To avoid heat rash, remove your sweaty clothes and jump right into the shower. Relieve the itchiness of the heat rash by applying a cooling mix of cornstarch and water.

Monsoon

The rainy season brings its fair share of skin problems, such as oily skin, open pores, boils, pustules, and rashes due to prickly heat. The heavily polluted atmosphere in cities can cause dust particles to cling to the skin, giving it a dull, grey appearance. Fortunately, frequent cleansing and freshening up of the skin can help keep it looking and feeling clean.

How to Protect Your Skin in Monsoon?

To take care of your skin during extreme humidity, those who easily suffer from prickly heat should regularly consume cooling drinks. To combat greasy skin and open pores, wash your face three times daily with a mild face wash. Rinse off every trace of soap with warm water, then cold water, and apply a toner.

Even if your skin is well balanced or slightly dry, it may be a good idea to switch to a lightweight moisturiser, one formulated for oily skin, which will feel less cloggy.

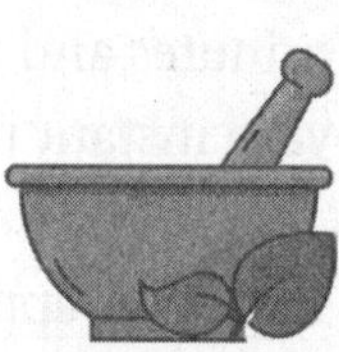

DIY Recipes to Protect Your Skin in Monsoon

Recipe 1: Try this special skin cleansing powder. Take 1 tablespoon of green gram powder, 1 tablespoon of Bengal gram powder, and 1 teaspoon of fenugreek seed powder. Mix

1 teaspoon of this powder with rose water and apply it on your face daily.

Recipe 2: Every night, drink a glass of water mixed with a crystal of rock salt and half a lemon juice. Use the other half of the lemon in your face mask—mix it in 1 teaspoon of honey and egg white. Apply it every day for 6–8 weeks for a remarkable improvement in your skin.

During the rainy season, when there is profuse sweating and the body is not exposed to air, red pustules the size of mustard grains may appear on the body, particularly on the chest, back, abdomen, and forehead. This can also cause itching.

Recipe 3: To avoid prickly heat and soothe the skin, dust the body liberally twice a day with equal quantities of boric powder, sandalwood powder, and talcum powder.

Recipe 4: Mix Multani mitti with water to form a thin paste and apply it to the affected areas. Once the paste dries, take a cold bath. Applying yoghurt to the affected areas before bathing can also help relieve prickly heat.

Recipe 5: To reduce inflammation in its early stages, apply kala jeera (black cumin seed) ground in water to the infected areas.

Recipe 6: For frequent occurrences of infected pimples on the face, apply neem tree bark ground in water in which neem leaves have been boiled.

Recipe 7: Mixing grated onion with sandalwood powder and applying it to the face helps cleanse septic pustules and makes the skin soft and smooth in a few weeks.

Maintaining healthy skin year-round requires adjusting your skincare routine to the changing seasons. This involves using the right SPF for sun protection, moisturising to prevent dryness, and making season-specific adjustments. By understanding your skin's needs and modifying your routine accordingly, you can keep your skin healthy and radiant in every season. The tips and recipes mentioned in this chapter are here to guide you through all the seasonal changes.

7
Decoding Your Ingredients

Most of the ingredients mentioned in this chapter are usually used in the form of a serum. You can either use these serums alone or combined with toners, facial oils, moisturisers, or creams. Serums are formulated to penetrate the deeper layers of the skin, whereas moisturisers and creams mainly target the upper layers. By using both serums and moisturisers in your skincare routine, you can provide your skin with complete benefits. It is important to stay consistent with this routine for a few weeks before evaluating the results, as both short-term and long-term improvements can be expected.

Unlike moisturisers, serums have an absorbent texture and an oily consistency that imparts radiance to the skin, enhancing its visual appearance. These can be used as a quick and convenient way to revitalise and enrich the texture of your skin, providing instant suppleness.

Here are some of the active ingredients that you can consider including in your skincare routine, depending on your specific skin concerns.

Vitamin C

Vitamin C serves as a natural shield for the skin, playing a vital role in producing collagen. As an antioxidant, it actively counteracts detrimental free radicals generated by factors such as pollution, stress, and poor diet. These free radicals can harm the skin, leading to premature ageing. Thus, the inclusion of vitamin C in both skincare creams and a balanced diet is crucial to ensure optimal skin health.

Squalene

Squalane is a versatile and beneficial ingredient in skincare that can be incorporated into a variety of products such as moisturisers, serums, and facial oils. It is a moisturiser emollient that functions like our skin's natural oils and keeps it healthy. When applied topically, squalane has some incredible skin benefits. It creates a protective barrier on the skin that prevents moisture loss. It's lightweight, non-comedogenic, and non-greasy, meaning it can moisturise without feeling heavy on the skin. Squalane intensely boosts hydration, making our skin look soft and supple. It is also a natural antioxidant that helps delay visible signs of ageing.

Niacinamide

While choosing skin products for the daytime, include products that are specifically formulated with elevated levels of vitamin B, particularly niacinamide, to cater to your skin's needs. Niacinamide, a vital nutrient for skin health, aids in minimising dehydration, enhancing collagen production, reducing pore size, and promoting an optimal level of fatty acids. Including Niacinamide in your skincare can have a positive impact on your skin's overall well-being.

Hyaluronic Acid

Hyaluronic acid is a natural substance in the body, mainly

found in connective tissues like the skin, joints, and eyes. In the skin, it retains water and maintains hydration, which can promote a healthy, youthful look. Hyaluronic acid serves as more than just a revitalising and renewing skincare product. It also effectively delivers other beneficial ingredients to the deeper layers of the skin, where they can have a more potent impact. Go for creams and anti-ageing products that contain hyaluronic acid to harness its benefits. Furthermore, hyaluronic acid helps plump and hydrate the skin, but it is not recommended for use around the delicate eye area.

Alpha Hydroxy Acids (AHAs)

AHAs are commonly present in various anti-ageing products, which are natural 'fruit acids' derived from plants. These organic compounds are recognised for their ability to gently exfoliate the skin and stimulate the production of fresh collagen—promoting firmer and more supple skin. Additionally, AHAs work by dissolving the adhesive bonds that hold dead skin cells together through washing or cleansing. This process encourages the skin to grow more cells, increasing cell turnover younger, contributing to a more youthful appearance. Make sure to apply sunscreen when using products containing AHAs as they increase the sensitivity to the sun.

Some common AHAs to include in your skincare routine are:

a. Lactic Acid: It provides enhanced moisturisation to the skin. It aids in retaining the moisture supplied by creams and lotions, making it particularly valuable in anti-wrinkle and anti-ageing products. These formulations effectively support skin hydration and promote a more youthful appearance.

b. Glycolic Acid: Derived from sugar cane, glycolic acid is known for its effective exfoliating and skin-brightening effects.

c. Mandelic Acid: It is derived from almonds and is gentler on the skin, making it suitable for acne-prone skin.

d. Citric Acid: Found in citrus fruits, it is used in skincare formulations for its exfoliating and skin-brightening properties.

Beta Hydroxy Acids (BHAs)

BHAs such as salicylic acid, aid in the removal of surplus skin cells through their chemical exfoliating properties. Additionally, they possess anti-inflammatory properties that help unclog pores, remove excess oil, and reduce redness, inflammation, and puffiness, resulting in smooth and calm skin. Compared to AHAs, BHAs are milder and can be used to address acne-related concerns.

Retinol

Retinol possesses the ability to reduce fine lines and wrinkles by promoting skin regeneration in the deeper layers. It is a form of vitamin A, which aids in the shedding of the upper layers of the skin while stimulating the production of collagen and elastin. Through these mechanisms, retinol effectively works towards improving skin texture and reducing the visible signs of ageing.

Kojic Acid

Kojic acid and arbutin serve as natural alternatives to hydroquinone, effectively targeting hyperpigmentation within the skin's layers. These compounds work by balancing melanin levels, thereby assisting in the reduction of hyperpigmentation. Their successful track record includes fading age spots, freckles, and sunspots, making them valuable options for individuals seeking to address such skin discolouration issues.

Alpha-Lipoic Acid (ALA)

Alpha-lipoic acid, also known as nature's potent anti-inflammatory and antioxidant remedy, surpasses the effectiveness of vitamins alone in promoting skin healing and hydration. Its remarkable power makes it an exceptional choice for enhancing overall skin health.

Essential Fatty Acids

Essential fatty acids (EFAs) are key ingredients in creams and lotions that greatly enhance skin health. With their non-greasy texture and oil-producing properties, EFAs can effectively plump the skin and prevent dryness. Products with EFAs provide nourishment while maintaining skin balance and hydration.

Ginseng

For ages, ginseng has been used as an herbal supplement or tea to enhance energy levels and alleviate inflammation in the body. However, in skincare, its primary purpose is to invigorate and rejuvenate the skin by promoting blood circulation, reducing puffiness, and providing a wealth of phytonutrients. Ginseng offers a holistic approach to skincare by effectively toning and revitalising the skin.

Vitamin Cocktails

The latest approach to enhancing skin with essential vitamins is to combine all the necessary vitamins for apt skin health into a single formula. By cleverly blending these vitamins, the skin's ability to absorb them is enhanced, resulting in improved efficacy and effectiveness of the creams. Some components found in vitamin cocktails are:

a. B5: Vitamin B5 is known for its function in aiding tissue repair, contributing to smoother and more youthful skin. It addresses concerns in the deeper layers of the skin, effectively preventing blemishes and fine lines. For best results, consider using it in conjunction with niacinamide, which can further enhance overall skin health.
b. Magnesium: It greatly diminishes the visibility of fine lines and wrinkles. This mineral aids in tightening the skin's surface while stimulating a new generation of skin cells. As a result, magnesium is frequently included as a component in age-defying polishers.
c. Zinc: When seeking minerals that enhance the skin, zinc emerges as the top contender due to its direct impact on skin regeneration from within. It proves beneficial not only for problematic and ageing skin but also imparts a healthy radiance while banishing dullness. By incorporating zinc, your skin can appear to be glowing, boosting its overall vitality.

Incorporating these ingredients into your skincare routine can be beneficial for your skin's overall health and appearance, as they can help address common skin concerns such as acne, hyperpigmentation, and fine lines. By using them in moderation and with the right products, you can achieve clearer, brighter, and healthier skin.

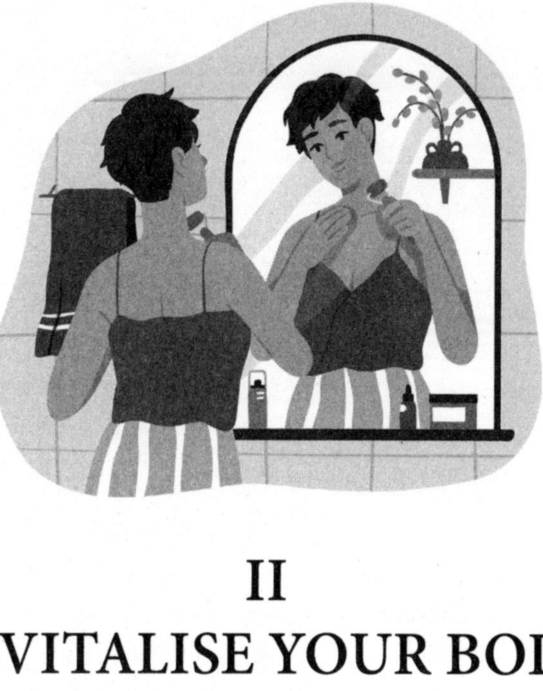

II
REVITALISE YOUR BODY

8

Nurturing Your Body

Beauty is always considered the sum of what you are and what you have. It cannot be restricted to only your face. You need to care for your body as well. Taking care of your body is important for staying healthy and feeling good. It not only helps you look better but stay strong as well. As we age, some parts of our bodies can become weaker if we don't exercise them enough.

Taking care of your body encompasses much more than just skincare or facial treatments. It's about nurturing yourself, inside and out, to promote health, vitality, and radiance. Let's delve into some aspects of holistic body care along with some DIY recipes to make you feel and look your best.

Care While Bathing

Taking care of your body while bathing is an essential part of maintaining good hygiene and promoting overall well-being. A proper bathing routine involves more than just cleansing; it encompasses a series of steps to nourish the skin, maintain hydration, and promote relaxation. By adopting mindful practices and selecting the right products, you can transform your bathing experience into a rejuvenating ritual that supports your physical and mental health. Read on to explore key steps to help you effectively care for your body while bathing, ensuring that each session leaves you feeling refreshed and revitalised.

Relaxing Bath

If your daily routine involves standing or sitting for long hours, it's not uncommon to feel exhausted at the end of the day. Your muscles may feel tense and tired, and you might find it challenging to unwind and relax. Taking a warm bath before bed can help rejuvenate and relax your body tissues. It can help soothe sore muscles, reduce inflammation, and promote better blood flow. The warmth of the water can also help calm your mind and relieve stress and tension, making it easier for you to fall asleep and get a good night's rest.

Recipe: Fill a bathtub with warm water. Add 2–3 handfuls of Epsom salt and 2 drops of lavender essential oil. Mix it properly.

Soak yourself in it for 20–30 minutes, relax, and end with a cold shower.

Body Polishing Exfoliator

This exfoliator is good for body polishing, nourishing, and rehydration. However, it is not recommended for sensitive skin.

Recipe 1: Take 2 tablespoons of white rice powder. Add 1/2 cup of plain yoghurt, 1 teaspoon of honey (or glycerine, if allergic to honey), 1 tablespoon of almond oil, and squeeze a few drops of lemon juice and 2 drops of lemon essential oil.

Mix it properly and massage it gently all over your body. Rinse it off with regular water. This paste will help remove dead skin cells, making your skin look radiant.

Recipe 2: Take 1/2 cup of grated coconut, add 1 tablespoon of almond oil, 5 drops of sandalwood essential oil, and 1/2 cup of yoghurt.

Mix all the ingredients and massage this paste gently all over your body. Wash it off with regular water. This scrub will help get rid of the dead skin and condition and moisturise your body as well.

Beat the Summer Heat

All you need is this cooling pack to keep your body cool, hydrated, and protected from the scorching heat. This pack is especially for those who spend a lot of time in the sun, as this helps cool the body while moisturising it.

Recipe: Take 1/3 cup of cucumber and add shredded mint leaves. Add 1/2 cup of aloe vera gel and 3–4 drops of lavender essential oil. Blend all the ingredients and refrigerate it for 20 minutes.

Apply this paste across your face and body, leaving it on for 20–30 minutes. Rinse it off with regular water.

Body Polish

This body polishing recipe deeply nourishes and brightens the body.

Recipe: Take 3 tablespoons of sesame seeds, 3 tablespoons of almond oil, 1 tablespoon of honey, and squeeze a few drops of lemon juice. Mix all the ingredients and apply them all over your body to make it look smooth and shiny.

Establishing wellness routines can be a proactive approach to managing common body problems and promoting overall well-being. We will now delve into some of these wellness routines and more home-made recipes.

Neck

A beautiful neck, like good skin, is not merely a gift of nature. Often, the neck, which is an extension of your face, is neglected and ends up wrinkled, with a crepe-like texture.

Common Neck Issues

- Dark patches, wrinkles, pigmentation, and dullness are caused due to a neglected skincare routine in the area.
- The neck and eyes age faster compared to other areas.
- Once the skin on your neck is wrinkled, rejuvenating it is difficult. Your neck responds slower to treatments than any other feature, except for the eyes. Be patient and persistent.
- Wrinkles on the neck appear due to the gradual drying of the skin and age-related sluggish metabolism.
- The blood supply to this area is particularly lax, resulting in rough, dull, muddy, or discoloured skin.

Hacks for a Beautiful Neck

- Regular exercise, massage, a thorough skincare programme, and a good posture lead to a beautiful neck.
- Extend your regular skincare regime of cleansing,

toning, and nourishing to your neck for a flawless complexion.

- When bathing, scrub your neck with a rough, soapy washcloth or a dried tori scrubber. Scrubbing will activate the circulation and remove every trace of deeply embedded grime and dirt.
- Always cleanse your neck both morning and night with good cleansing milk. Also, make sure to properly remove make-up before rinsing.
- Once a week, use a fine scrub to remove dead skin cells as you do for your face.

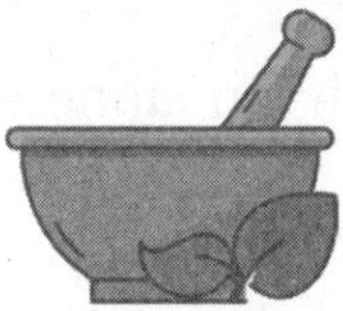

Home-Made Recipes for Your Neck

For Dryness

Recipe: You can make a scrub at home by mixing 1 tablespoon of sandalwood powder, 1 tablespoon of Multani mitti, and enough yoghurt to make a paste. Apply this and rinse it off after ten minutes.

For Nourishment

Recipe: Good skin food for the neck could be made with equal quantities of cold cream, almond oil, and rose water.

To massage the neck, first apply some cream on the fingers of each hand. Then, clasp the base of the neck with your thumbs in front and your fingers meeting behind.

Gently massage from the bottom upwards, until you reach the ears. This will help to relieve tension in the neck and promote relaxation.

For Dullness

Recipe: Revitalise your lacklustre neck skin with rejuvenating and firming masks. Mix 1 tablespoon of dry oatmeal powder with yoghurt and add the juice of one lime.

Gently massage this pack on your neck and leave it in for half an hour. Rinse off, pat dry, and apply a moisturiser. This mask will help remove the dead skin cells, and the lemon j uice will aid in restoring the acid balance while also bleaching the skin.

Follow this up with an almond oil massage for the best results.

Back

A flawless back is every woman's dream. Backless dresses or dresses with a deep back look best when your back has a healthy glow. To achieve this, it is important to take care of your back just like any other part of your skin.

Back care involves cleansing, exfoliating, and moisturising. Additionally, some exercise is important to maintain a great looking back. However, your back can be prone to various problems such as excess oiliness, acne, blackheads, pigmentation, tan, and dark patches.

Back Care Routine

a. Cleansing: This is the most important step to begin your back care routine. Dampen your back, pour some face wash or body wash on a handle brush or a loofah, and gently brush your back to unclog the pores and remove sweat and grime. Do this every day.

b. Scrub: The aforementioned brush will have done some part of the scrubbing, but you need to whip up a home-made scrub to get of rid eruptions and blackheads to have a glowing back. You can use oatmeal, rice flour, or even sugar scrubs. Add a few drops of essential oil, such as lavender or patchouli, to the scrubbing element of your choice. Honey also acts as a great moisturising component to add to your scrub. Keep the scrubbing gentle. Do this twice a week.
c. Moisturise: Of course, it is important to moisturise your back. Use a good body lotion or body cream (for dry skin) and let it set in well.
d. Sun Protection: Use sunscreen regularly to avoid damage to your back, especially if it is exposed. Remember to use sunscreen especially when you are stepping out, going swimming, or hitting the beach.

Hacks for a Beautiful Back

a. A Toned Back Is a Sexy Back: It is not possible to target specific areas of the body for fat loss, however, we can tone and define muscles through exercise. To strengthen and define your back muscles, focus on exercises that target this area. Furthermore, pay attention to your posture, try to pull your shoulders back and stretch your spine. This will help to ensure that your back muscles are both toned and strong.

b. Regular Massage: Of course, the daily cleansing and moisturising work, but for a flawless back, visit a spa. A regular massage and some packs will do wonders.
c. Natural Bleach: Many women opt for chemical bleach for their bodies. I have always propounded the use of natural bleach for your face and body, and I would recommend the same for your back, too. Go for a protein bleach that naturally lightens your skin by getting rid of the tan.

   Mix milk powder, lemon juice, honey, and papaya and apply the paste on your back for 20 minutes for a natural bleach. Wash it off with regular water.
d. Don't Forget the Shimmer: When you are out for an event and your back is showing, don't forget to use make-up. Apply some moisturiser and sunscreen and follow it up with a foundation. To add an *oomph* factor, mix in some shimmer in your foundation.

Chest and Abdomen

Most women are extra critical about their breasts—too big, too small, wrong shape, sagging—it is never perfect. Regardless of your breast size, a good posture goes a long way to give you a great form. It is worth noting that individuals with smaller bust sizes have a unique advantage—they do not have to worry about the effects of gravity on their breasts, which can help maintain a youthful appearance for a longer period.

On the other hand, women with larger busts need to take extra care to support them and ensure they remain shapely and firm. Unfortunately, many women with larger breasts resort to poor posture, such as stooping with rounded shoulders, to try and hide their bust size. This not only fails to flatter their overall body shape, but it also causes their breasts to droop over time.

Here are a few ways you can exercise your breast muscles:

a. Try this exercise to improve posture. Stand in your usual position. Now, lift the shoulders slightly, move them back about two inches, and drop them from this point, so that the back and shoulder muscles lift the pectorals and, in turn, the breasts, extending the areas from the navel to the diaphragm, which improves the bust line.
b. However out of condition your breasts are, they can always be improved with exercise. The most efficient bust conditioning sport is swimming. The breaststroke is best, as the name suggests.
c. Exercises to strengthen your bust can be done at any moment during the day. Here are three exercises for lifting your breasts.
    - Sit cross-legged or on your heels, in Vajrasana, and extend your arms behind you, interlacing the fingers. Hold the position for a count of 10 and then relax. Repeat 3–4 times.
    - Sit on the floor or a chair and lift your arms overhead, pressing the palms of the hands together. Using your muscles and still pressing your palms against each other, lower them slowly to shoulder level. Count to 10, relax, and repeat.

- Clasp hands and push hard against each palm. Relax and repeat when you have a spare moment.

4. Massage your breasts every day, as it also helps the lymph move and reduces the risk of breast cancer. Place your finger between the two breasts and massage in an upward and outward stroke. As you move your fingers, your palms will firmly massage the breast. Then move your palms to massage downwards on the outer sides, and your fingers will meet below the breast and bring them up again. Repeat the motion at least 30 times.

How to choose the right bra?

Many women wear the wrong size bra, which is problematic because proper support is necessary. Here is a sizing guide: Measure your circumference directly under the bust and add five inches. That is your bra size. If a second measurement around the fullest part of your bust is the same as the bra size, you need an A cup; if it's 1 inch more, a B cup; if 2 inches more, a C cup; and if 3 inches more, a D cup.

A bra that is too tight for your back can cause pressure marks under the arms and mid-back. Straps that are too tight leave ridges on the shoulders, and ill-fitted cups can accelerate mastitis (inflammation of the breasts).

Hacks for a Beautiful Abdomen

- Stretch Marks: Stretch marks occur when the skin cannot stretch to accommodate rapid growth during puberty or pregnancy. Prevention is key. If you are pregnant, try lubricating your tummy with a vitamin E-enriched cream or oil to avoid getting stretch marks. Don't let your skin become dry.

  - To make stretch marks less noticeable, apply a touch of waterproof make-up with a damp cotton pad in a shade that matches your skin tone.

- Better posture: A straight back helps to pull in the belly.
- Firming Gel: Apply the firming gel on your tummy and wrap it tightly with cling wrap. Leave it on for 30 minutes. This will help reduce bloating and water retention.
- Eat Slower: Eating quickly makes you store excess fat in your belly.
- Drink Lemon Water: To boost metabolism, drink a warm glass of lemon water in the morning.
- Apple Cider Vinegar: Consuming small amounts of apple cider vinegar also helps to promote fat loss.

Legs

Having smooth and flawless legs can get you all the attention you seek. While you can turn to quick hacks for a last-minute party, there is nothing like a consistent leg care routine to ensure that your legs are always fabulous and luminous.

Hacks for Beautiful Legs

- Massage your thighs while bathing. Gently knead and massage the area, as this leads to improved circulation.

With a soothing motion, cleanse the skin with soap, gently twisting and pressing to invigorate the flesh. Afterwards, pat dry and apply a nourishing body lotion.

- If the skin on your knees tends to get dark and dry, make sure to apply a moisturising cream. Also, once a week, massage them with a mix of 1 tablespoon of oil (any oil), juice of half a lemon, and half a teaspoon salt before you bathe.
- Legs tend to be dry compared to other body parts due to the lack of active oil glands. Thus, moisturising after a shower is essential. Consider applying a hydrating body cream or lotion to replenish moisture.
- Spider veins, which are often around the knees and thighs, are not something that can be neglected. Proper medical treatment is important. It is also beneficial to rest as often as possible with your legs raised. Furthermore, applying cypress essential oil to the affected areas can be helpful.

Remember, true beauty radiates from within, reflecting a harmonious balance of physical health, emotional well-being, and self-love. By prioritising holistic body care practices, you can enhance your natural beauty and cultivate a profound sense of vitality and confidence.

9

Cellulite: Strategies for a Smooth Body

Cellulite is a combination of excess fat, water, and extracellular waste, which becomes lodged in the connective tissues of our body. Once the cellulite is trapped, it pushes up against the network of the skin's restraining fibres, appearing as unevenly distributed lumps and pads of fat on our body.

Cellulite is different from the ordinary layer of fat that lies beneath our skin. Unlike cellulite, the evenly distributed fat layer provides insulation and cushioning to the internal organs, serving as a source of energy. The tendency to develop cellulite is largely hereditary, affecting both young and old, men and women alike.

Where Can You See Them?

Women are more likely to have cellulite in the prominent areas of their bodies, with excess fat deposits typically found on their breasts and hips. In men, excessive fat deposits are often found on the abdomen and upper back, around the shoulders and neck.

Causes of Cellulite

- Most cosmetologists agree poor diet, poor physical maintenance, internal stress, and inadequate elimination are the primary causes of cellulite formation. Food poisoning also causes cellulite.

- A sedentary work life and lack of physical exercise lead to improper elimination and excess retention of the toxic cellular waste (lactic acid) in our muscles. This promotes the build-up of new cellulite.
- Excess sodium consumed as common salt leads to the retention of water and a bloated feeling. As a result, it encourages the formation of cellulite.
- If our diet lacks adequate calories and nutrients or the food taken is hot and spicy, it results in irritation and aggravation of the digestive and intestinal tract. This produces stress within our bodies. This can further be worsened by poor elimination.

Ways to Control Cellulite

While eliminating cellulite may not be possible, there are several strategies you can try to reduce its appearance.

Diet

Eat sensibly to avoid stress and help the body cleanse itself of all irritating and polluting agents through the process of elimination. A wholesome diet should consist of four basic food groups—dairy, food, meat, vegetables, fruits, and cereals. A well-balanced and nutritious diet is efficacious in managing cellulite. Consulting a good dietician can also help in deciding the correct diet for your body type.

Controlled Fasting

Controlled fasting is an ancient system for cleansing and

resting the internal organs. Most individuals prefer a day of raw fruit juice fasting, while some opt for raw vegetable juice fasting. The power of vitamins, minerals, enzymes, amino acids, and other valuable detoxifying elements in the juice helps to work well without the interference of solid food. This is recommended for only one day per week.

Morning Fruit Cocktail

The fruit cocktail is prepared as follows:

Soak a cup of sun-dried apricots in pineapple juice overnight. Drink this cocktail first thing in the morning. The pineapple juice extracts the iron and copper from the apricot, which, in turn, enriches the blood with oxygen. This oxygen is required to awaken and revitalise the circulatory system.

Regular Exercise

Besides a balanced diet, one should follow a regular and planned exercise programme. It promotes a sense of well-being and reduces stress in our everyday life. It also helps eliminate waste materials within the body that otherwise contribute to cellulite.

Incorporating both cardiovascular exercise, such as running, swimming, or cycling, and strength training into your routine can help tone your muscles and i mprove circulation, which may reduce the appearance of cellulite.

A word of caution: One should not workout to the point of exhaustion that can have a negative impact. Therefore, avoid overexerting yourself.

Stiff Bath Brush

While taking a bath, after applying soap, scrub with a bath brush all over your body. This will help enhance blood circulation below the skin, which, in turn, will help get rid of the stored fatigue causing the build-up of lactic acids, carbon dioxide, and other chemicals.

Taking a shower with warm water before bed can also help steam out the accumulated toxins through the pores in the skin.

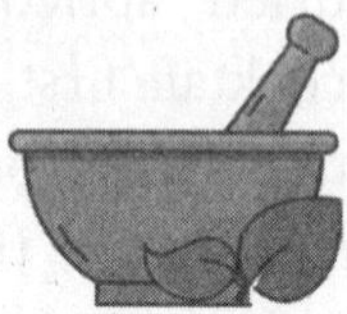

Home-Made Hacks for Smooth Skin

Recipe 1: Add two handfuls of Epsom salt in a tub of hot water. Soak in it for 20 minutes.

Recipe 2: Boil a handful of Ivy leaves and a handful of lotus leaves in about 1 litre of sesame oil for 20 minutes. Use this oil for massaging the cellulite areas daily.

Remember, consistency is key when it comes to managing cellulite, and what works for one person may not work for another. It's important to be patient and realistic about your expectations.

10

Nourishing Your Hands

Like your face, voice and eyes, your hands also express the real essential. There are some things you simply cannot hide, and your hands are a great example; they are your ambassadors to the world. It always seems a pity if they are neglected, as they let down your whole appearance. Nails, too, speak volumes about how much you care about your appearance.

Hard water, detergents, chemicals as well as skimping on hand drying can quickly lead to rough, dry skin, giving it a sandpaper-like texture. If you persist in using your nails and fingertips to rip open parcels and boxes as well as using them as tools to be used for jabbing lift buttons or dialling telephone numbers, you aren't doing your hands any good. If you've fallen by the wayside, read on, help is here.

One golden rule to follow for good-looking hands is to apply a good, lubricating hand cream after washing. Protection is the secret. Creams and oils do not soften the hands; they merely hold in the moisture in the skin and prevent its escape. Hand skin is just as vital to your appearance as well-groomed nails. For exposure to harsh chemicals and cold, dry air, the answer is protective gloves. For sunlight and sports enthusiasts, a sunscreen that contains Para-Aminobenzoic acid is crucial to screen out the ageing ultraviolet rays. Winds and long exposure to water call for petroleum jelly, which is an inexpensive and effective barrier.

A Handful of Issues

1. Rough or Chapped Hands: This is usually caused by the lack of vitamin B-complex. So, it's important for you to take a course of tablets or injections. Additionally, try a compress of an infusion of marigold petals for chapped or rough hands.
2. Sweaty Hands: This is the result of a sudden release of 'cold sweat' from the eccrine sweat glands. This is usually a nervous condition and the only remedy for this is to always carry a bottle of Eau De Cologne with you so that you can dab a few drops on your palms when needed. Also, it's beneficial to increase your intake of vitamin B-complex to get this issue under control.
3. Red Hands and Chilblains: Hands that suffer from inflamed, swollen red patches during winter need to try these exercises to improve circulation:
    a. Stretch your hands and fingers out in front of you as much as possible while keeping them tense. Hold this position for ten seconds and then slowly release the tension in your fingers. Repeat this exercise ten times every day.
    b. Shake your hands vigorously several times a day to improve blood circulation. Additionally, take a course of calcium tablets for stronger bones and massage your hands daily to relieve any tension or stiffness.

Nails

Nails are easier to understand when compared with hair, as both are primarily composed of dead tissue protein. Nails are considered healthy when you feel fit and maintain a well-balanced diet. Foods rich in vitamins A and B Complex, such as liver, citrus fruits, milk, honey, celery, cauliflower, nuts, and grapes are beneficial for the nails. Furthermore, vitamin D capsules can be particularly helpful.

Brittle and splitting nails are caused by a lack of calcium. This can be improved by taking two tablespoons of gelatine daily mixed in a glass of fruit juice. You can see results after six weeks. Ragged cuticles are caused by a lack of lubrication, so it's important to moisturise with plenty of cream. Ensure that both the cuticles and the area around the nails are well-hydrated to eliminate raggedness and hang nails.

Nail-biting is often a sign of anxiety and is also unsanitary. Self-discipline is the only solution to this habit. Try to approach life more calmly and maintain your nails. if your nails require strengthening as they grow, use a colourless nail hardener.

Manicure

A manicure once a fortnight can prove to be beneficial for an elegant appearance. Before every manicure, soak your hands in some warm olive oil for about five minutes. You can also try this home-made hand lotion to keep your hands soft and supple: Add 1/2 cup of rose water, 1/4 cup of aftershave, 1/4 cup of glycerine, and 1/4 tablespoon of white vinegar. Mix them well and apply them to your hands. Store it in a bottle for further use.

Here are some other tips you need to keep in mind:

- To shape your nails, use the smoother side of an emery board and shape them either oval, round, or square.
- Neglected cuticles tend to stick to the nail, so it's important to keep them healthy. To do this, apply some cuticle cream to your cuticles and push them back.
- Then, use a stick wrapped in cotton and dipped in cuticle remover to remove all the dead cuticle. If you have any hangnails, snip them off with a cuticle cutter, but do not cut the cuticle as it will only make it rough and hard and increase the chances of an infection.
- Once you're done with your cuticles, massage your hands with a good hand cream.
- To remove any residues from your nails, wash and dry your fingertips.
- Finally, apply nail polish.

Prioritising the care of your hands is essential for maintaining overall skin health. Regular moisturising, protection from harsh elements, and gentle cleansing are simple yet effective practices that can keep your hands soft, supple, and youthful-looking for years.

11

Navigating Foot Care

The feet are the pedestals of beauty. Your posture, your figure, the grace of your movement, and even the expression on your face depends upon your feet. You must have noticed the look of strain and misery of women whose feet hurt.

The human foot has 52 bones and 214 ligaments. It is subject to more pressure and injury than any other body part. Additionally, it can also be affected by a wide variety of diseases, circulatory disorders, dermatitis, diabetes, and arthritis.

However, minor foot problems often stem from external pressure and everyday complaints, such as corns, calluses, and ingrown toenails. These issues are painful and could worsen without timely attention and proper treatment.

Some Common Feet Problems

1. Corns and Calluses: Corns and Calluses are caused by the ways we walk and due to friction. To get rid of these, it is to better walk barefoot or wear comfortable footwear whenever possible. A massage with olive oil or castor oil also helps soften the dead tissues.

   Try these tips:

   a. A salt foot bath followed by a massage with lemon peel oil can feel soothing. You can make this by turning half a lemon inside out and filling it with olive oil or any other vegetable oil. Allow the oil to steep overnight.

b. To ease the pain of corn, tape garlic or onion on it.

c. Rubbing a pumice stone over calluses, which have been softened while bathing, reduces them and eventually eliminates them.

2. Itchy Feet: Lemon juice and vinegar applied to the feet can prove to be beneficial in controlling itchy feet.
3. Athlete's Foot: It is an infection caused by a fungus that leads to rashes between the toes, often along with minute blisters splitting the skin. Apply some onion juice between the toes to relieve itching.
4. Cracked Heels: Mix 100 grams of coconut oil, 5 grams of camphor, and 20 grams of paraffin wax. Melt and store this in a tin. Apply this mixture on clean feet at night every day till the cracks disappear. Additionally, wash your feet in the morning and moisturise.
5. Ingrown Toenails: They are mostly self-inflicted by incorrect trimming of the nail, cutting too short, or snipping down the sides, which can tear the nail and result in a sharp piece piercing the skin. To heal the wound, new skin is formed and builds up. One should see a chiropodist at the first sign, as in severe cases, the whole nail may have to be removed. Always cut to enails straight across and avoid cutting corners back into the groove.

6. Swollen Feet: Swelling can be caused due to various reasons. Make sure to apply both hot and cold compresses to the feet.
    a. Lie or sit with your legs elevated and soak your feet in a tub of hot water and add a handful of Epsom salts as well as a handful of normal salt.
    b. You can also tie crushed leaves of geranium over your feet to reduce the swelling.
    c. Using cedarwood oil is a good remedy for swollen feet. You can either add 2 drops to a tub of water to soak your feet or you can add 1 drop to a carrier oil and massage your feet with it. Be careful to not use excess.

7. Perspiration of the Feet: It's crucial to not suppress it, as severe and incurable diseases may follow and persist until the feet perspire again. Instead, use a foot powder: Take 1 1/2 cups of talcum powder, 2 tablespoons of boric acid, 1/2 cup of cornstarch, and mix these ingredients together. Apply it to your feet.
8. Chilblains: This occurs due to poor blood circulation, exacerbated by cold, damp weather. Scratching an itchy chilblain can worsen it, potentially causing a break that requires medical attention. However, if the chilblains are unbroken, applying iodine ointment at night can be helpful to an extent.

   If you are prone to chilblains, it's important to keep your feet warm and engage in foot exercises. Alternating between bathing your feet regularly in hot water followed by cold water can assist in better circulation.

Lastly, adding a bit of pepper to your foot powder and sprinkling it in your stockings can help alleviate cold feet.

Can Your Feet Give You Wrinkles?

Yes! Every time you squeeze into a shoe that's too small and wince from pain, you create an unpleasant facial expression that could stay with you for a lifetime. It isn't worth it. Feet can easily be made happy and pretty.

Always try on shoes in the afternoon on a hot day. At this time, your feet are as big as they're going to get, so you can't be fooled into buying the wrong size. Since everybody has one foot larger than the other, try on both shoes before you buy them. If the shoe is uncomfortable, try another style.

Avoid wearing high heels for long periods of time. For extended standing durations, use sturdy leather-lined shoes with a broad-based medium heel. Don't use the same pair day in and day out. Leather loses its shape unless allowed to rest for a day or so.

To exercise your feet, occasionally, move around barefoot. Walking on sandy beaches and thick grass stretches your arches and makes your toes work. Alternatively, you could walk on a carpet for 30 minutes. Also, picking up marbles with your toes can improve the state of your feet. Lastly, spare some time once in ten days to give yourself a pedicure.

12

Removing Unwanted Hair

In many societies, there is a prevailing perception that facial and body hair on women don't align with conventional beauty standards. As a result, some women undertake regular efforts to manage such hair they may find undesirable.

Furthermore, many women also suffer from excessive body hair, also known as hirsutism, which is often influenced by genetic factors. Variations in hair density can also be observed among different ethnic backgrounds. Individuals with darker hair might feel particularly self-conscious about excess body hair, as it tends to be more noticeable compared to lighter hair tones.

Causes of Excess Hair

The overactivity of the endocrine glands during puberty, menopause, or due to certain internal disorders can lead to the growth of superfluous hair. During puberty, hormonal disturbance is characterised by erratic menstrual cycle, underdeveloped breasts, and often hairiness. Stress and anxiety also contribute to excessive hair growth. Emotional stress and anxiety disturb hormonal activity, which stimulates the hair follicles in our body.

Certain drugs can adversely react and cause hirsutism. Drugs most likely to cause hair growth include birth control pills, cosmetic creams containing hydrocortisone—a drug to dry up milk glands in new mothers—and dilantin—used for epilepsy.

Tumours or cysts of the ovaries, diseases of the adrenal glands, malfunctioning and tumours of other endocrinal glands, such as the pituitary and thyroid glands, can also lead to a serious hormonal imbalance that triggers hair growth.

Methods to Remove Extra Body Hair

Several methods can be used to deal with excessive and unwanted hair. However, here, we will discuss the methods that people can easily follow at home.

Shaving

It is the quickest and easiest method to follow, but it must be done more frequently than any other method. For the best results, shave regularly, as often as once or twice a week.

The misconception that shaving with a razor makes hair grow coarser is wrong. Shaving only leaves an oblique tip, which feels coarse until the sharpness wears off. Never dry shave with a razor. If your skin is sensitive, apply some almond oil or moisturiser. Then lather with soap or shaving cream for a closer finish. Use long, upward strokes on the legs and under the arms. While shaving, the top layer of skin is loosened, so using deodorants immediately after shaving can cause irritation. If hair regrowth starts early, smooth it with a pumice stone.

Bleach

This method is extremely useful for concealing light, fine, and fuzzy hair. However, bleaching is not recommended on very dark hair, which tends to turn yellow-orange in colour. When done properly, bleaching is both safe and simple.

There are certain skin types that are sensitive to bleaching agents, so always perform a patch test. First, apply a little bleach to your neck and wait for 20 minutes. If there is no reaction, go ahead.

It's important to note that bleaching can sometimes damage the hair shaft and cause temporary breakage.

Tweezing

It is one of the most popular and effective methods used to remove scattered hair on the face, such as around the eyebrows. Plucking out hair has no adverse side effects as is the case with other methods of temporary hair removal.

Some points to remember:

- Constant and repeated tweezing leads to tiny pits and scars
- It is important to sterilise the tweezer to avoid infections
- Do not pluck hair from moles and warts
- Rub some ice on the area before and after tweezing to ease the pain

Waxing

This method is ideal for legs, arms, and underarms. Post waxing, hair typically reappears in about 4–6 weeks. The more the areas are waxed, the less is the hair likely to regrow as it damages the hair follicles. Hot wax is the best for removing facial hair, which is applied to the area, allowed to cool a bit, and then pulled off in the opposite direction.

Make your own wax at home: Take 500 grams of sugar, 1 cup of water, 1/4 teaspoon of citric acid, and 1/2 tsp of glycerine. Boil the water and sugar till the sugar melts. Then, add citric acid, which has been dissolved in 1/2 cup of warm water. When it reaches one thread consistency, remove it from the stove and add glycerine.

Depilatories

These chemical substances remove unwanted hair by dissolving it from the skin's surface. Depilatories are available in the form of creams and liquids. Before using them, wash and dry the area to be depilated. Apply the cream and leave it on for as long as specified on the box. Then, wash the area with soap and water and pat it dry. Follow it up with a moisturising lotion. Often, new hair growth appears in a week.

Note: It's important to follow the instructions carefully when using depilatories to avoid skin irritation or adverse reactions.

Taking care of the skin on your feet is crucial for your overall well-being. By regularly cleansing, moisturising, and exfoliating, you can prevent common issues such as dryness, cracking, and infections. It's also important to wear comfortable shoes and practice proper foot hygiene to maintain healthy skin. Keep in mind that healthy feet contribute to your overall comfort and mobility. So, prioritise their care to maintain optimal foot health and quality of life.

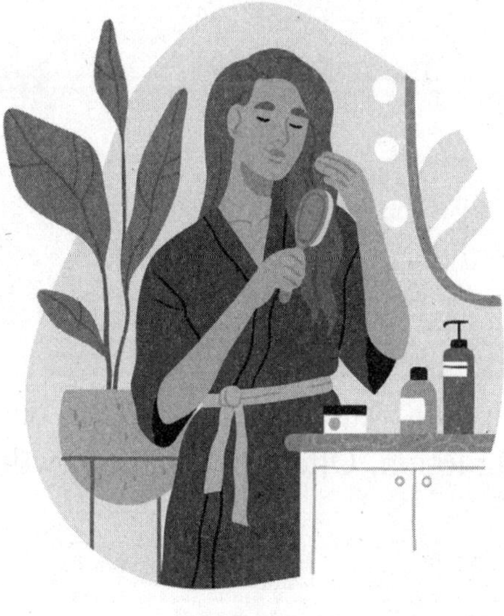

III
NOURISHING YOUR LOCKS

13
Hair Care 101

Hair is an essential part of our appearance and personality, and it is also one of the most versatile accessories we have. Healthy hair can be a wonderful permanent asset that complements our style, accentuates our fashion appeal, and frames our faces. It is a fluid medium of self-expression and art that allows us to express ourselves in a unique way.

However, maintaining healthy and vibrant hair requires more than just occasional grooming. It demands a deeper understanding of its complex nature and distinctive needs. Like any other aspect of self-care, effective hair care begins with knowledge—knowledge of the composition, structure, and behaviour of our hair. By understanding hair a bit more, we can make it easier and more effective to maintain it.

From nourishing treatments to styling techniques, each aspect of hair care contributes to the preservation of its beauty and resilience. This section will help you embrace a holistic hair care approach, transforming it from a mere accessory into a radiant expression of your true self.

What Is Hair Made of and How Does it Grow?

Hair consists of strong, elastic strands of protein called keratin, and in chemical terms, it is composed of oxygen, iron, nitrogen, hydrogen, sulphur, carbon, and phosphorous.

The exact proportions of these chemical elements vary with sex, age, type, and hair colour.

The sources of hair are very small, tiny pockets in our skin and scalp known as follicles. Follicles are not spread evenly on the scalp but are found in groups of two to five each. Every follicle follows a life cycle of its own, producing six inches of hair a year, for as long as four years, before it falls out, then starts all over again after a short period.

During the active period, the new cell growth pushes the older part of the hair away from the papilla until the hair falls out. It is the pattern of cells grown at the papilla that determines whether the hair growth will be straight, wavy, or curly.

The growth pattern usually becomes uneven during adolescence when hair growth is at its peak, gradually declining as we grow older. Additionally, the cell growth pattern can also change due to illness, certain drugs, or pregnancy.

Although a hair strand looks like a singular fibre, each strand comprises three different layers—the cuticle, the cortex, and the medulla.

The cuticle is the outermost layer of the hair, which protects the inner cortex. It consists of flattened, hard, dead cells. When the cuticle breaks and dislodges at the end of the hair, it leads to split ends. Improper care and frequent use of harsh chemicals on hair can also damage the cuticle.

The second layer is the cortex, which is composed of fibres twisted together like a rope. The qualitative properties of strength, elasticity, pliability, growth pattern, width, and texture of hair depend on the composition of the cortex. It provides hair with its colour. The presence of the four natural pigments—black, brown, yellow, and red—are logged in the cortex in varying proportions. The air spaces in the cortex determine the colour and shade of the hair.

Lastly, the innermost layer is called the medulla, which is composed of soft keratin. The medulla may not be present in some hair, resulting in a very fine texture.

Some of the most common characteristics of healthy hair are:

- Thick and dense
- Fine and silky—not too oily or rough
- Shiny and glossy
- Flexible—capable of setting and styling
- Full-bodied and not limp

Factors Affecting Hair

The health of one's hair reflects their overall health and well-being. Apart from improper hair care, several other factors can negatively impact the condition of hair.

Some of those factors are:

- Genetics
- Chemical and drug reactions
- Hormonal changes
- Emotional stress and trauma
- Illness
- Improper nutrition

These factors, by and large, influence hair condition and its proper growth, which we will examine in detail while discussing the different hair woes in succeeding chapters.

Types of Scalps and Hair

Scalps can vary in characteristics such as oiliness, dryness, or sensitivity.

Oily Scalp

When the oil glands present in the scalp secrete excess oil, it travels down the hair shaft, causing excessive oiliness on both the scalp and hair strands. Oily hair appears lank, dark, and coarse.

Dry Scalp

Dry hair is a result of the lack of natural sebum and oil production, causing the hair to dry out at a cellular level. Flakiness of the scalp and dandruff are a direct result of dryness. Dry strands look limp and rigid, making them more susceptible to breakage and damage.

Normal Scalp

A normal scalp is healthy, with silky hair—without dry ends or excessively oily roots. This kind of scalp is the easiest to care for.

Combination Hair

Combination hair is a condition when the roots of your hair become oily, while the ends remain dry. This happens because the natural oils don't reach the end of the hair. This condition is often caused due to using the wrong type of conditioner or styling products, exposure to humidity and pollution, and very long hair.

How to Check Your Hair Type

Wash your hair and let it dry normally. The next morning, part your hair and run a tissue along the scalp. If it appears to be greasy and has a slight stain or discolouration, it means you have an oily scalp. If the tissue appears to be dry, wait for another day and repeat the test. If it still looks dry even after 3–4 days, you have a dry scalp.

Your Go-to Hair Care Routine

Taking care of hair is much the same as taking care of your skin. An effective hair care routine involves regular cleansing, toning, and conditioning. Another important aspect of efficient hair care is the use of proper products, as different types of hair require different hair care products. Keep in mind that using incorrect products can damage your hair.

Oiling

Regularly oiling your hair is essential for maintaining its health. Oil not only nourishes your scalp and strands but prevents brittleness as well. Furthermore, oiling helps increase blood circulation to the scalp, promoting hair growth, while forming a protective barrier on the strands.

To oil your hair, take 1/2 cup of olive oil, add 2–3 curry leaves, 3 peppercorns, 1 pod of garlic, and 1 tablespoon of castor oil. Heat all the ingredients in a pan. Cool down the mixture and add 2 drops of tea tree essential oil, 2 drops of rosemary oil, and 2 drops of lavender essential oil. Apply this mixture to your scalp and strands for beautiful and stronger hair.

Toning

To tone, gently massage your scalp. This action helps in stimulating blood circulation, which is required for healthy and strong hair. This is not a full-blown head massage; it is only about teasing the scalp with your fingertips by applying gentle pressure. You can tone your scalp without using any product. If you want to, you can use a hair toner, a mild hair oil, or a blend of essential oils. Spend at least 3–4 minutes to stimulate your scalp. Shampooing your hair after this process is entirely up to you.

Cleansing

Regular cleansing of the scalp is necessary to maintain overall hair vitality and health. A good shampoo helps remove dirt and product build-up without stripping your hair of natural oils.

There are shampoos with special ingredients to it to make your hair look and feel healthy and shiny. Use different shampoos to determine what suits you the best hair.

What Makes a Good Shampoo?

A good shampoo removes dust, grime, and build-up from your scalp while nourishing the strands. If you are not using a gentle shampoo, dilute it with equal quantities of water and then use it to wash your scalp and hair. Keep in mind that if you directly apply a harsh shampoo to your scalp, it will leave a residue, causing flakiness and hair fall.

You can use pH-balanced shampoo daily if it won't strip off natural oils or hair colour. You also must use a detoxifying shampoo once in two weeks to get rid of the stubborn dirt and product build-up that coats your hair over time. As these shampoos contain enzymes and AHAs, they help to deeply cleanse your scalp and hair.

Lastly, ensure that you thoroughly rinse your hair post-shampoo to remove any trace of the product.

Conditioning

The most important part of hair care is conditioning your strands. Conditioning is a restorative routine that helps nourish your hair when it becomes excessively stripped of moisture or oil due to the usage of harsh shampoos, overexposure to the sun, or the application of harsh chemicals such as perm lotion, straightening lotion, regular blow-drying or straightening, or excessive hair colouring. The routine will restore and correct the imbalance.

The type of conditioning required depends on the physical health of the hair. I have dedicated a complete chapter to this topic.

Balancing Act: Managing an Oily Scalp

A proper hair routine is required that aims at removing the excess oil and exfoliating skin cells that clog up, suffocating the hair follicles. This blockage of follicles can also lead to several infections, which can further cause hair loss and other scalp disorders.

Follow a customised cleansing and toning routine. Since the hair must be washed as frequently as it gets dirty and oily, a mild and natural shampoo is ideal for an oily scalp.

Massaging your scalp is also important for the overall well-being of your hair, which promotes healthy growth. For oily hair, massage with a toning lotion and follow a two-minute brushing, stroking, and combing routine.

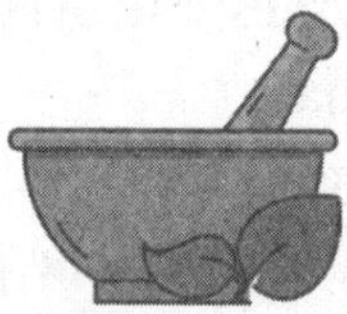

DIY Care for Oily Hair

Below are some simple yet effective recipes that work wonderfully for an oily scalp.

Cleansing Pack

Recipe: Powder some green grams and fenugreek (*methi*) seeds. Mix two portions of shikakai powder, one portion of green gram flour, and half a portion of fenugreek powder. Mix this powder with water to make a paste and apply it to your scalp and hair. Rinse it off after 30 minutes. This mixture won't lather like a typical shampoo but will cleanse your hair.

Natural Shampoo

Recipe: Take some dry soap nuts (*reetha*) and soak them in water overnight. Mash them in the morning and strain the soapy solution. Add 1 teaspoon of shikakai powder to it and wash your hair with this mixture.

Shampoo Infusion

Recipe: Boil two handfuls of mint in 1 1/2 glasses of water for 20 minutes. Strain this solution and add in a 300 ml bottle of your shampoo.

If you are unable to make your cleanser at home, mix this concoction in your shampoo for the best results.

Toning Lotion

Recipe: Mix 1 tablespoon of malt vinegar or apple cider vinegar in a glass of water. Add a pinch of salt to it.

Dab 2 tablespoons of this mixture on your scalp and massage it with your fingertips twice a week. Leave this toner for one hour before rinsing it with cold water. You can then brush and set your hair.

Combatting Dry Scalp: Essential Care Strategies

Dry hair tends to be thin and brittle, making it susceptible to tangles, damage, breakage, and split ends. The primary aim of a dry hair routine is to replenish the oil and moisture. Apart from genetics, a harsh cleansing routine and dry toning and massaging of the scalp can cause dryness and flakiness.

Often, a generous application of oil or a hot oil massage is recommended before washing the hair. Also note that frequent shampooing can cause more harm to your already dry hair, resulting in excessive hair fall.

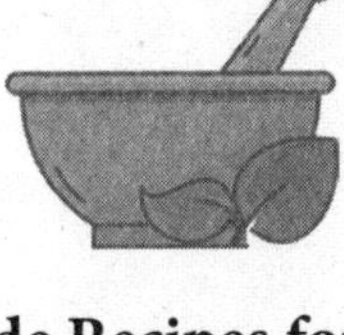

Home-Made Recipes for Dry Hair

Below are given few natural recipes that are time-tested. For maximum results, use these recipes regularly in place of chemical products.

Gentle Cleanser

Recipe: Take 1 cup of coconut milk and add 2 tablespoons of gram flour or 1 teaspoon of shikakai. Massage this gently into your scalp and hair. Leave it on for 5 minutes before rinsing your hair. Use this cleanser at least once a week.

Protein Conditioner

Recipe: Beat 1 tablespoon of castor oil, 1 tablespoon of glycerine, 1 teaspoon of apple cider vinegar, and 1 teaspoon of protein. Add 1 tablespoon of mild herbal shampoo as well. Apply this to your scalp and leave it on for 30 minutes. Shampoo hair with warm water.

Massage Oil/Toner

Recipe: Take a tablespoon of coconut/olive oil and add 1 teaspoon of castor oil and 3-4 drops of lavender essential oil. Heat it a little and massage it gently into your scalp and hair. Leave it overnight and shampoo your hair in the morning. Repeat this routine at least once in two weeks.

It is important to understand your scalp and hair needs before following a routine, so you can cater to them better.

14

The Importance of Conditioning

Our hair suffers from the effects of modern lifestyles, where the air is polluted and the water is laden with chemicals. Moreover, to make matters worse, we often resort to using strong products containing harsh chemicals, hoping they will solve our hair woes. All these factors contribute to split ends, dryness, extreme oiliness, and limp or frizzy hair. But worry not, as this is where the conditioner comes to your rescue.

A conditioner is a beauty product that enhances hair texture and makes it easily manageable. This is achieved through the action of positively charged polymers, both small and large cationic molecules, present in the conditioning agents. These molecules attach to the negatively charged damaged areas of your hair. As a result, each hair shaft is coated and protected, which can aid in repairing weakened hair. Conditioner is an essential step in the shampooing process.

Modern conditioners are formulated to penetrate much deeper into the hair shaft, compensating for any deficiencies in lustre, gloss, and moisture, thereby leaving the hair better conditioned.

Why Using a Conditioner Is Important

Conditioning is an essential aspect of hair care, and almost all types of hair need it. It rejuvenates our hair which is typically robbed of its vitality because of external damage.

Conditioning is, in fact, a restorative routine and falls in the category of preventive hair care:

- Restores Body and Bounce to Limp Hair: There are two kinds of body-building conditioners—the ones you rinse out and the ones you leave in. Both work at adding bulk to the hair by leaving some material on the hair shaft. These materials include polymer fibres and proteins.
- Restores the Acid Mantle: The special cream rinse conditioners are designed to untangle the frizz in the hair. Many also add the welcome beauty benefits of high gloss to the locks.
- Restores Damaged Hair: Deep conditioning treatments help to restore dry, damaged hair, plus hair that is brittle excessively and broken in any way. The deep conditioners contain large amounts of protein. For these proteins to be absorbed, the deep conditioner should be applied for a longer time.
- Restore Moisture Loss: Conditioners also help in reducing friction and adding combability to hair. Additionally, they help in removing dryness and moisturising it.

Hair Masks

Hair masks work on the same principle as conditioner, except they are left on the hair for a longer time and penetrate the hair deeper. These ingredients are absorbed by the hair, so we do not have to leave them on longer than recommended. Use a hair mask once a week and apply a hot towel over it. I prefer doing this as the extra heat and steam prevent the hair from drying out, resulting in super glossy hair.

I also find that using cold water as the final rinse leaves the hair shiny as it closes the cuticles. It also promotes hair growth by stimulating blood flow to the scalp.

Leave-in conditioners simply nourish and add shine to the hair without leaving it limp. They are excellent for people with fine, fly-away, or difficult-to-manage hair. They should be applied from the roots.

The Conditioning Prescription at Glance

Frizzy and Unmanageable

Cause: Humidity

If anyone has frizzy and unmanageable hair, it is often caused by high humidity levels. To tackle this issue, using a moisturising cream conditioner can work wonders. The conditioner helps to hydrate and nourish the hair, reducing frizz and making it more manageable. By adding cream conditioner to your hair care routine, you can combat the effects of humidity and enjoy smoother, healthier-looking locks.

Limp, Flat, Brassy

Cause: Sweat

Perspiration, a weak acid, takes the life out of hair. Wash it out as soon as you can with a mild shampoo. For treated hair that turns brassy, try a colour rinse. Add 1 teaspoon of instant coffee to your conditioner before use.

Faded and Dry Hair

Cause: Overexposure to the sun

Faded and dry hair can be attributed to overexposure to the sun. To combat this, it is important to take preventive measures. Wearing a hat can shield your hair from direct sunlight while using hair sunscreen provides an extra layer of protection. These precautions help prevent the sun from stripping off moisture from your hair, keeping it healthier and less prone to dryness.

Greenish and Brittle Hair

Cause: Chlorinated pools

Greenish and brittle hair is often caused by exposure to chlorinated pools. Chlorine and metals can be absorbed by the hair, leading to a change in hair colour. To fight this, you can use a soda-water rinse to help remove chlorine residue. To reduce dryness, it is recommended to give your hair an oil massage once a week. Using a swimming cap can also provide a protective barrier for your hair.

Dull, Limp, and Unmanageable Hair

Cause: Pollution

Dull, limp, and unmanageable hair can be attributed to pollution. Dirt and pollutants in the air can cling to the hair, causing it to lose its vitality. To counteract the effects of pollution, you can create a solution by mixing 1 mug of water, 6 ml of rose water, and 4 ml of vinegar. Apply this mixture to your hair and rinse it out after shampooing. Use this twice a month. Additionally, using fewer hair products overall can help minimise the impact of pollution on your hair.

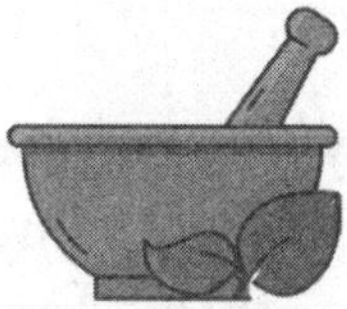

Home-Made Hair Conditioners

There are several easy DIY conditioner recipes. These are not as harsh as the chemical conditioners but are effective.

The All-Purpose Moisturiser

Recipe: Mix 1 teaspoon of castor oil, 1 teaspoon of Amla/Brahmi oil/olive oil, 1 teaspoon of malt vinegar/apple cider vinegar, 1 teaspoon of glycerine, and 1 teaspoon of shampoo.

The castor oil provides body to hair, the herbal oil acts like a hair tonic, vinegar restores the acid mantle, glycerine moisturises the hair, and shampoo is the medium that blends the ingredients.

Before washing the hair, apply the mixture and leave it on for about 30 minutes. Shampoo and condition and feel the marvellous change in your hair texture.

For Shine and Sheen

Recipe: Grate a few onions and some cabbage together and cover them in a copper utensil overnight. In the morning, add a few drops of ylang-ylang essential oil to remove the smell of onion. Add a few drops of herbal oil and then apply it to your hair. Shampoo after 30 minutes. Your hair will gain a superb gloss and colour. You can follow this routine once a week.

Henna Conditioners

Recipe 1: If you have oily hair, mix henna with 2 tablespoons of yoghurt and a pinch of sugar to make a light paste. Add a bit of water if the paste is thick. Apply this to your hair and leave it on for 30 minutes.

Recipe 2: If you have dry hair, mix henna in 1 tablespoon of oil and warm milk to make a paste. Apply and leave it on for 30 minutes.

These henna conditioners will provide colour, sheen, and body to your hair.

Hair-Setting Conditioner

Recipe: Mix 1 teaspoon of gelatine and a few drops of ylang-ylang in a mug of water. Rinse your hair with this concoction. Air-dry your hair and set it as you desire.

To Reduce Hair Fall

Recipe: To prepare a natural hair mask, take half a cup of grated coconut and add warm water to it to make coconut milk. Alternatively, you can buy it from the market. To this, add 1 teaspoon of honey, 1 teaspoon of malt vinegar, and 2 drops of rosemary essential oil. Mix everything well and apply it to your hair. Leave it on for half an hour. Rinse it off with water and follow up with a natural shampoo and conditioner.

Conditioning from Within

What we eat and drink is reflected in how we look and feel, including the state of our hair. Simply using good quality shampoos and styling agents cannot enhance hair appearance. You must improve its condition by nourishing it from the inside.

Zinc, protein, iron, and vitamins A, C, and B12 are essential ingredients for healthy hair. Lack of any of these can lead to extreme hair loss. It's important to maintain a balanced diet, and equally important to hydrate your body with 6–8 glasses of water daily. Improper eating habits and crash diets can be detrimental to your hair because the body perceives this as an emergency and shuts down the delivery of nutrients to non-essential body parts. The first thing to suffer is your hair, followed by your skin and nails. Stress, anxiety, and sleeplessness have the same effects. Consult your doctor for a supplement if this is a regular occurrence.

Calcium and magnesium are also necessary, and you can obtain them from milk and its products. A glass of warm milk with turmeric or saffron before bedtime can be helpful. If you are a vegan, you can get calcium and magnesium from green leafy vegetables, which help reduce stress and control anxiety and fear. Additionally, chamomile tea is better than regular tea as it soothes the nerves.

Eating salads and vegetables like broccoli, cauliflower, and cabbage is great for your hair. Jatamansi is used for relaxation and promoting good sleep.

Massage a few drops of lavender and orange blossom mixed with vegetable oil and water into the scalp to calm any stress or anxiety.

15

Conquering Dandruff

Dandruff is the most common problem that individuals face at least once in their lives. Having a few white-flaked cells is normal, as it is the scalp's way of shedding dead skin cells and waste material through the pores. It only becomes a problem when you experience an excessive build-up of these white flakes. Properly maintained, clean, and healthy hair with the right acid balance does not face this issue.

There are two kinds of dandruff—oily and dry. Dry dandruff appears as loose, white flakes, which come along with a great deal of itching. On the other hand, oily dandruff is sticky and yellow in colour, and the scalp has an unpleasant smell. The oily form is found most among adolescents and adults who have excessively oily skin and scalp.

What Causes Dandruff?

Dandruff can be caused by a variety of factors, such as:

- Improper diet
- Anxiety
- Hormonal imbalance
- Fungal infections
- Scalp injury

- Unwise or excessive use of hair products
- Dry weather

Getting Rid of Dandruff

The key to hair care is to keep it clean. Wash your hair and scalp frequently; this could be daily or every other day, depending on how stubborn your dandruff is. If your hair and scalp are oily, you should opt for an herbal shampoo, since washing your hair frequently with a strong shampoo can damage it.

Wash your hair and scalp with a mild anti-dandruff shampoo. As most anti-dandruff shampoos are quite strong, I suggest diluting them with water.

Daily massaging and brushing are extremely helpful in treating dandruff. They boost blood circulation to the scalp, promote the flow of oil, and dislodge dead skin cells sticking to the scalp, making exfoliation easier. If you have dry dandruff, consider using an oil to massage your scalp, especially before washing your hair.

Consume animal fat, polyunsaturated vegetable oils, nuts, chocolates, fried foods, shellfish, and iodised salt in moderation. Follow a diet high in green vegetables, lean protein like chicken, fish, and yoghurt, and foods high in vitamins A, E, and B-complex.

Lastly, ensure that your combs, clips, bands, and rollers are cleaned regularly and that your pillow covers and towels are changed frequently. Do not share your combs and brushes with anyone.

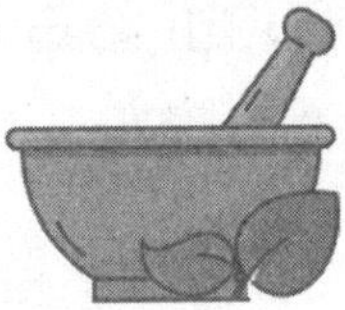

DIY Recipes to Cope with Dandruff

Dandruff can be easily taken care of with some simple home-made recipes.

For Oily Dandruff

Triphala Lotion

Recipe: Buy some triphala from the market. Mix 1 teaspoon of it in a glass of water and boil this mix. Let it simmer for about three minutes. Cool and strain it.

Mix 2 drops of lemon essential oil and add equal quantities of apple cider vinegar or malt vinegar. Gently massage this lotion into the scalp. Use this every night, and cleanse with a mild shampoo in the morning.

Vinegar Rinse

Recipe: To a mug of water, add 2 tablespoons of malt vinegar and 2 drops of rosemary essential oil. After shampooing, rinse your hair with this concoction.

This is an excellent remedy to prevent oily dandruff.

A Dandruff Cleanser

Recipe: Soak 2 spoonfuls of methi seeds in water overnight. In the morning, make a paste of these seeds and add a squeeze of lemon juice. Apply this on your scalp and leave it on for half an hour.

Then, wash your hair with soap nut (reetha) or shikakai and water. Use this twice a week.

Hair Pack

Recipe: In half a cup of sour yoghurt, add a squeeze of lime and 3–4 drops of patchouli essential oil. Massage it into the scalp and leave it for 30 minutes before washing your hair.

For Dry Dandruff

Oil Massage

Recipe: Massage your scalp with 1 teaspoon of hot castor oil mixed with 1 teaspoon of coconut oil, 1 teaspoon of sesame oil, and 2 drops of lavender essential oil. Leave it on for 30 minutes before rinsing it out with shampoo. Follow this routine twice a week, especially in winter.

Hair Pack

Recipe: In 5 tablespoons of yoghurt, squeeze half a lime and mix in 2 spoonfuls of green gram powder. Apply this mixture to your scalp and leave it on for 20 minutes. Then, thoroughly wash your hair with a creamy shampoo. Follow this routine at least once in a week.

If the dandruff does not clear up in time, you must consult a doctor.

16

Coping with Hair Loss

Like everything else, hair, too, has a life cycle. Each hair strand that grows must fall out one day, with a new strand sprouting up at the same place. There exists a natural balance between the rate at which hair falls and new hair grows. Any imbalance in the body can lead to issues such as excessive hair loss or hair growth all over the body. Unfortunately, nowadays, hair loss is a common problem that may occur due to various reasons such as:

- Emotional and physical stress of city life
- Local scalp infection
- Adverse drug reaction
- Hormonal imbalances during puberty and/or pregnancy
- Poor diet

Interesting Facts about Hair Loss

Over the past several years, dermatologists have made some interesting findings that explain the pattern of hair loss. Curiously enough, the phenomenon of falling hair is related to the rate of hair growth, length of the hair, age and even the colour of hair.

a. It is normal to shed about fifty to eighty strands of hair a day. It is normal for each of those strands to be replaced by the hard-working follicles. On any given day, about 90 per cent of hair is in the growing stage. This period lasts for about 1000 days. 10 per cent of hair is in the resting stage, which lasts for about 100 days before the follicles eventually grow out.
b. Interestingly, the fall out occurs mostly in the morning. The cause, however, remains unexplained.
c. The length of hair is an important factor in hair loss. The 4-inch-long hair loses an average of 87 hairs a day; the 12-inch-long hair loses about 26 hairs a day, and 20-inch-plus long hair loses as few as sixteen hairs a day on average. The longer the hair, the less hair loss there is.
d. Hair typically grows 6 inches a year, and a shortfall in normal hair growth is often accompanied by hair loss, too. Apart from the day-to-day loss, we shed more than usual hair during six periods of our lives—from birth to age three, at ten, at twenty-two, around the age of twenty-six, at thirty-six, and around fifty-four. This occurs due to hormonal changes that take place in our bodies during these periods.
e. For women, the maximum hair growth occurs between the ages of fifteen and thirty.

Causes of Excessive Hair Fall

Technically, an unnatural excessive hair fall, temporary or permanent, is called alopecia, which is caused by reasons as explained below.

Hereditary

The kind of hair we have—whether thick, thin, fine, sparse, straight, or curly—depends a great deal on the genes inherited. The problems concerning hair loss are also passed on from the parents to the offspring. Diabetes and thyroid disorders are two real threats to healthy hair.

Trauma

The result of physical stress on the hair is called traction alopecia. This can be caused by tightly tying up the hair in chignon styles, ponytails, or braids. Prolonged and continuous pulling or pressure on the hair can result in spot baldness. Spot baldness can also occur due to trauma or sudden shock, like a severe blow to the head.

Local Scalp Infection

Bacterial, viral, or fungal infections can cause hair to fall out in spots. However, these infections can be treated with medicated shampoos and lotions.

Diseases

Internal disorders and infections that can cause high fever, such as flu, pneumonia, typhoid, etc., are often accompanied by excessive hair loss.

Chemicals or Drugs

Antibiotics and a drug called Cortisone, administered sometimes in treating acne and scars, can lead to hair loss. Chemical therapies given for serious diseases such as cancer can also cause excessive hair fall.

Emotional or Environmental Stress

People who are unable to cope with the pressures of life, constantly worrying about problems at the workplace or home, and have unresolved emotional conflicts, are susceptible to excess hair loss. Tension can cause the muscles in the scalp and neck to constrict, obstructing blood circulation and resulting in the suffocation of hair follicles. To prevent extreme hair loss, massaging the scalp to loosen it up can prove to be effective.

Pregnancy

Generally, the condition of the hair improves during pregnancy as the endocrine glands function at their peak. Hair loss typically occurs only after the birth of the baby due to irregularities in the functioning of the thyroid glands. This can be attributed to lifestyle changes associated with caring for a new baby. Normal hair loss after delivery typically begins four months after birth and continues for about two months.

Birth Control Pills

If a woman in perfect health, with normal weight, regular menstrual cycle, healthy eating habits, and physical activity, uses birth control pills for contraceptive reasons, she can experience hair loss problems. Taking the pills can alter the hormonal balance. However, if a woman already suffering from hormonal imbalance takes the pill, it can restore balance and promote hair growth.

Menopause

One of the problems of menopause is the slowing down of the production of the female hormone, oestrogen. This can result in weak, dry hair and excessive hair loss in one out of two women.

Ways to Prevent Excess Hair Fall

Hair, in normal and healthy conditions, does not fall out at an alarming rate. The excess hair fall mostly occurs when the hair is extremely dry, rough, and damaged. Conditioning and nourishing aid in preventing excess hair loss. Cream helps rinse the dry and rough hair and regain its flexibility. A generous application of moisturisers and oil replenishes the moisture in dry hair.

Massage is another important element of scalp treatment for controlling excess hair fall. It invigorates blood circulation, providing hair with an increased supply of nutrition and oxygen for healthy growth. Furthermore, massage also stimulates dormant hair follicles to grow fresh hair.

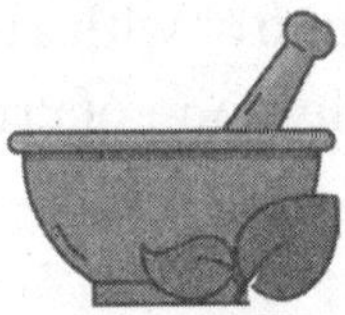

DIY Routine to Manage Hair Loss

Try these age-old recipes to control excessive hair fall:

Hair Rejuvenating Ointment

Recipe: Take 10 grams each lime seed powder and black pepper powder. Make a fine paste in plain water or, if possible, in ginger juice. Apply this paste to your scalp every day. Massage it in using your fingertips for 5 minutes. Leave it on for at least a couple of hours before rinsing it out.

For Bald Spots

Recipe: Make a paste with *mulethi* (liquorice) powder and milk cream. Add a little saffron and apply it on the bald patches at night. Massage the bald spot generously with your fingertips for 5 minutes as you apply this ointment. Leave it overnight and wash your hair in the morning.

Oil Massage

Recipe 1: Castor oil is an excellent ingredient for hair growth. Just add 2 drops of rosemary essential oil to it, part your hair in small sections, and apply the oil with cotton. Massage it in with your fingertips.

Recipe 2: Squeeze the milk out of half a coconut, add the juice of half a lime, and 2 drops of lavender essential oil. Massage into the scalp and leave it on for 4–6 hours. Wash your hair either with a mild shampoo or with a paste of crushed hibiscus leaves mixed with 1 tablespoon of crushed fenugreek seeds.

17

Navigating the World of Hair Colour

Many of us are concerned about maintaining a youthful appearance, and for some, the appearance of grey hair can be undesirable. However, it's important to note that grey hair is not solely grey but a mix of white and brown, creating the illusion of grey.

The appearance of grey hair doesn't always correlate with age; it can manifest even in younger individuals, while some fortunate people never experience it. Typically, grey hair starts to appear in one's thirties as the body naturally produces less pigment.

Nobody wakes up with grey hair overnight. While factors like shock or illness might temporarily affect the production of pigment, it's only when new hair grows that the grey is visible.

For those who prefer not to dye their hair, choose softer colours in clothing and make-up to complement the natural changes in skin tone that accompany ageing.

Temporary Hair Colour

In this treatment, the hair shaft is coated with a clear colour to darken or highlight it. If you are not going to fight the greys, the temporary rinse will keep it looking bright. It's temporary, as you are only coating each hair strand until the next shampoo. Colours are available in coloured conditioning setting lotions, water rinses, and shampoos, enhancing grey hair with silver, pearl, or blue tones.

A rinse can also add burnished gold or copper highlights to light or medium-coloured hair, bringing out the red tones and brightening dark hair with shine.

Semi-Permanent Treatment

Semi-permanent hair colourant shampoos come in one bottle and require no mixing. They penetrate the hair slightly and do not need the help of a peroxide developer. The resulting hair colour fades gradually and naturally, lasting through four to six shampoos. As the colour fades, there is no need for root retouching. However, most semi-permanent colours will only conceal up to 25 per cent of grey hair. They blend white hairs into your natural shade but usually do not completely cover them. The key to success is choosing a colour as close to your own as possible. Semi-permanent colouring is relatively easy to do at home. The results are very natural, and the colour does not transfer onto linen or clothing. Touch-ups are unnecessary because a new application is repeated every four weeks.

Permanent Hair Colour

If you have a lot of grey hair, only a permanent colourant will completely cover it. Look for packs with two bottles to mix. One contains colour, the other peroxide, which helps the colour penetrate deeply into the core of each hair to give a longer-lasting colour—six to eight weeks—and the biggest colour change. You can even lighten your hair. Most are shampooed on, and the colour doesn't wash out. However, after about every four weeks, the roots will need retouching. Modern applicators make it easy to apply the colour just where you want on the roots—where the new hair growth is showing.

The disadvantage of oxidation colouring is that it makes the hair dry and porous, so use plenty of conditioners. The hair colourants now available in the market are ammonia-free. Ammonia is a strong alkali used to make the colour compound penetrate deeply. But colourants formulated without it are less likely to irritate the skin, do not smell as strongly, and leave the hair in better condition.

Today, there are two kinds of permanent hair colouring products available—penetrating tints and coating tints, like herbal hair dyes.

The subtlest way of camouflaging grey hair is to have streaks done professionally. Tiny, thread-like sections of hair are tinted all over the head, and as hair is made up of several different shades, results can be very natural-looking. Less retouching is necessary.

Hair Colouring Techniques

There are several hair colouring techniques, and each offers unique effects and results. Below are some of the most popular ones.

Money Piece

Money pieces focus on lightening the area around the hairline, creating a face-framing effect. The money piece technique adds a pop of colour and vibrancy to your hair while accentuating your hair colour and facial features. It's basically like a highlighter, for your hair.

Root Smudge

In this hair colour technique, your colourist will leave your roots a little darker than usual and seamlessly blend your roots with your chosen hair colour so that when your hair grows out, it looks natural.

Ombré

This technique melts darker roots into brighter ends. It's a lot more obvious than balayage because there's no definition of natural colour through the ends. Ombré is also more dramatic as it requires fading between two different shades of hair dye.

Babylights and Ribbon Highlights

Both babylights and ribbon highlights are a subtler version of highlights. The sections of hair are smaller, which creates a look that's just as dynamic but less bold than regular highlights. In babylights, thin highlights are placed at your roots and around the edges of your face. Whereas ribbon highlights have thin highlights woven into the lengths of your hair, adding small hints of colour throughout.

Sombré

A sombré is a subtler version of the ombré technique that fades between two colours closer in tone.

Balayage

It is a low maintenance, 'lived-in' style that's subtle but can be built up over time. It's perfect for when you're ready to hit refresh but don't want a major change. It works on most hair types and colours and can transform a solid colour into ribbons of different shades.

Foilayage

Foilayage is a combination of balayage with the use of foils, more often seen in the traditional application of highlights, to create brighter, lighter sections throughout while retaining a natural-looking finish and seamless blending.

How To Choose Hair Colour

Now that you know the methods to change your hair colour, the most important point is determining the colour that's correct for you. You can't just make a blanket statement and say, 'I want my hair to look the way it did when I was twenty-five.' When you were twenty-five, your dark hair looked right with your complexion. A quarter of a century later, however, that same near-black hair will be much too harsh for your skin and face and will make you look older.

The rule to follow is—the darker your hair colour, the younger you should be; the older you are, the lighter your hair colour should be.

How Often to Colour Hair?

The primary rule is to avoid overlapping of colour by retouching surfaces every four weeks. No more, no less. If dyeing or bleaching is scheduled sooner, you overprocess the previously treated hair, which becomes quite noticeable from the hair's dry and brittle appearance. If you bleach or colour your hair within five or six weeks of a previous treatment, it can result in an uneven hair structure.

This is harmful since the original chemical process of dyeing or bleaching alters the structure of the hair to begin with. So, an exact four-week retouch is a must. Additionally, after colouring, you must allow your hair to remain dry for three days and three nights to allow the process to oxide properly.

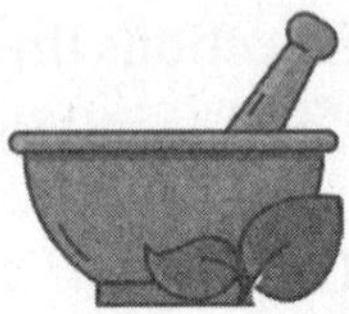

Colouring Your Hair at Home

With Henna

Recipe 1: You can make different shades by using henna powder. Mix 2 cups of henna powder in 1 cup of warm water to make a thick paste. Add 1 teaspoon of lime juice to help release the dye. Let it stand for one hour. Adding 1 tablespoon of ground cloves for a darker shade

Recipe 2: A dark brown shade may be obtained by mixing one part henna with three parts of indigo.

Recipe 3: Mix 1 tablespoon of coffee and 2 tablespoons of amla powder mixed with henna. This can also help darken the hair.

To counteract the drying action of these mixtures, add curd and 1 tablespoon of raw mustard oil.

With Walnut Shells

Recipe: Walnut shells make another harmless dye that progressively adds colour to the hair.

Place walnut shells in a mortar and cover with water. Add a touch of table salt. Let it stand for 3 days. Now add 3 cups of boiling water and simmer for 5 hours, always making sure that the evaporated water is replaced. Extract the dark liquid from the shells using a press or by twisting the shells in a cloth. Replace the separated liquid in the pot again and now reduce it to a quarter of its volume. Add a small piece of alum as a fixative. At first, it will produce a somewhat yellowish effect, but it will finally give the hair a deep black colour. Remember to use this on shampooed hair.

With Tea

Recipe: Boil 4 teaspoons of any tea in a quart of water until a very dark brown liquid is obtained. Use alum to set the dye. Strain and use this concoction like a rinse. Repeat rinses until the desired shade is acquired.

Rules To Remember for At-Home Colouring

1. Always do a patch test: This is extremely important especially when you are using a market product for the first time. Use a cotton ball to remove any natural oil from behind your ear or in the crook of your elbow and then apply a dab of the colouring product. If you experience any breaking out or itching within 24 hours, take an antihistamine, drink plenty of liquids, wash

the experimental area off well, and throw out the stuff! Don't skip this important step as allergic reactions can be devastating.

2. Work with dirty hair: Always use hair colour or bleach on hair that hasn't been cleaned in a few days. It's incorrect to shampoo it first, contrary to directions on most do-it-yourself products. The natural oil protects your skin against the unwanted invasion of chemicals into the system. Don't even brush your hair the morning before colouring it.
3. Don't fight the red in your hair: Amateur colourists make the mistake of trying to eliminate any red pigmentation. However red pigment is an important factor in the actual structure of the hair. If you try to remove this colour via over-tinting or bleaching, you remove the last link that holds the chain reaction of the hair together. Especially for dark hair, more red highlights look flattering, so exploit them, don't eliminate them.

Some Colouring Tips

- Leave your highlighting and creative colouring to professionals.
- Use a shampoo and conditioner specially formulated for coloured hair to prevent colour from fading. Acid balance shampoos and conditioners help lock in the colour pigments and improve the condition of the hair.
- For dull and faded colours, there are two quick home remedies. Mix 2 tablespoons of protein powder with

milk and apply it to your hair after shampooing, working it through your hair. Leave it on for 10 minutes and rinse thoroughly with lukewarm or cold water. Your last rinse should be a mug of water to which a few drops of ylang-ylang essential oil have been added.

- Another remedy for faded hair and to make your hair fresh, bright, and glossy, which I use a lot, is tea for brown hair and chamomile tea for blonde hair. Steep three tea bags in a large jug of hot water. Let it cool down and use it to rinse your hair. Chamomile solution is made in the same manner.
- Another natural remedy I use frequently is avocado. I use it when I have been in the sun and my hair feels dull, dry, and brittle. I mash up an avocado and work it through my hair after shampooing. I leave it on for ten minutes to let the moisturising oils penetrate the shaft and rinse it out.
- I will never forget the day I coloured my hair and went swimming. My hair turned green! That's when I discovered that the chlorine in the water can mess with your hair colour. Here are two after-swim hair recipes: Rinse your hair with soda. The second is to restore blonde hair to its original colour by massaging tomato juice into your hair after shampooing and rinsing out after five minutes. This helps to remove chlorine from the hair.
- We have talked about colouring, now let's talk about some fun colouring. Maybe put a contrasting colour around your face or dip the ends of your hair in a

bright colour. Believe me, it is a fun way to perk up dull hair.

- The semi-permanent colour lasts for a few washes—maybe twelve. With semi-permanent colour, you can only go darker and warmer, and it is mostly vegetable-based.
- Coloured mousse and gel are applied to the hair before it is set or blow-dried, changing your colour for the evening.
- Coloured wax and pomade are applied after the hair is dried and styled. When using coloured waxes, gels, and pomades, do a patch test, especially if your hair has been bleached or if you have blonde hair, to make sure it will wash out and not stay in the hair.
- Coloured hair mascara is wonderful for adding coloured streaks to your hair, and coloured spray is my favourite for adding some oomph and sparkle to your style.
- Since your hair is a canvas, techniques like dip-dyeing, tie-dyeing, tonal blasts, hidden colour, duo colour, and 3D effects can produce amazing results.
- My favourite is a personalised hair colour that complements the haircut.
- If you are scared to go in for colour, then ask your stylist to weave coloured hairpieces into your style.

18

Caring for Long Hair

Long hair needs special care, and when it isn't properly cared for, it begins to look like a rope left outdoors for months. Shampooing with the correct shampoo, specially formulated for long hair, is essential. After shampooing your hair, take extra care as wet hair is fragile and can break easily.

After washing your hair, don't brush it instantly. Instead, wrap it in a towel and blot out some of the moisture. Rubbing splits the ends and tugging very wet hair in its weakened state pulls out the hair. When your hair is slightly dry, comb it with a wide-toothed comb, starting from the ends and slowly working up to the crown. In this way, you avoid tangles and excess pulling.

A problem faced by many is an oily scalp, coupled with dry and split ends. Follow your shampoo with a final rinse of diluted vinegar—1 tablespoon of vinegar to a mug of water. This helps restore the acid mantle that has just been washed away. Also, use a good creamy conditioner only on the ends. Oily hair also requires brushing to keep oil from pooling on the scalp and to carry the oil to the hair ends to prevent the ends from drying out and splitting.

Brushing correctly with the right brush is probably the single most important factor in caring for long hair. Use a brush with natural bristles or with rounded synthetic bristles set in a back that is durable with a handle that fits comfortably in your hands. The best way to brush your hair, of course, is with your head hung down, while you brush finely from nape to ends of hair. Use firm, even strokes. Don't tear your hair and don't yank it.

Leading trichologists recommend frequent massage of the scalp. Massage certainly loosens the scalp and improves circulation, giving elasticity to the hair. Start massaging with the fingers together at the top of your head using the cushions, not the tips of your fingers. Make rotary movements, working over the entire scalp and moving the scalp, not the fingers.

Split ends, especially in long hair, are a result of rough treatment of your hair. Fierce brushing snaps the hair and breaks it off. The use of rubber bands to tie hair together, and winding hair into a fishhook with metal curlers or rollers can damage your long tresses. To avoid split ends, your hair deserves gentle, capable handling. First, trim the hair above the split ends. Keep them under control by using a cream conditioner on the dry ends. Don't use metal or wire rollers.

Girls who wear long hair in tight plaits and women who wear tight chignon seem to be the most frequent victims of spot baldness. It is caused by pulling the hair tightly back in an elastic band or bun in the same place for a long period. The position of a ponytail or a bun and the parting of these hairdos should be changed often if hair loss is to be avoided. Hair pulled back into confined styles should have the benefits of extra care in correct brushing and massage.

Once again, for those of you who use electric rollers, curling irons, and blow dryers, be sure to condition your hair after shampooing and use hot oil treatments regularly to keep hair from drying out.

Some Easy Hacks

A quick and easy way to put your hair up is by using a bun ring. You will easily find them in any accessory shop. A high ponytail never goes out of fashion and looks super sexy. Other classic styles that you will never go wrong with are a top knot, chignon, and French braids.

To prevent a harsh look while styling a bun, loosen some wisps of hair around the face. Always backcomb the roots of your hair for a firm foundation for your updo. I have always used accessories to make an instant change. If you are not too good with hairdos, accessories also help to cover up flaws and they can make any style look pretty.

I also use liquid tools to style long hair—gel, mousse, and spray. I love coloured mascaras to brighten up the hair. The colours I love using are gold and copper for highlights and bright blue and burgundy to add glamour. A glitter spray applied along the parting looks amazing for a special event. I have also found that rubbing a few drops of ylang-ylang essential oil between the palms of your hands and then down the hair not only creates shine but also adds an exotic aroma. Ylang-ylang is also an aphrodisiac that will create an aura of beauty around you.

Make sure to change your parting regularly. Try using a ponytail extension. Another way to add glamour to your hairdo is to pin your hair away from your face using a big silk flower or a jewelled clip. If your hair is too thin, fine, and silky to put up, first crimp your hair and then put it up. Crimping adds texture.

Don't wash your hair before doing an updo. It will make your hair difficult to handle. Ensure that the accessories that you use are not so heavy that they pull down your hair.

Lastly, avoid styles that are too difficult; try something easier. Messy hairstyles look casual and fashionable.

19

Chemical Treatments

Chemical treatments these days are professionally designed for the active, on-the-go lifestyle. There is a special chemical treatment for every individual, depending on the texture and type of hair. Each treatment should be customised to suit your unique hairstyle and lifestyle.

Successful restructuring of the hair necessitates the expertise of a professional hair designer. Their knowledge and experience are essential in determining what exact technique is required to create the look designed just for you.

There are myriad advantages of chemically treated hair. The finished look offers the wearer adaptability and versatility. The hair benefits from the support of a professional, both aesthetically and functionally.

Frequency of Permanent Waves or Hair Straightening

As the name implies, curling or straightening is permanent. As the hair grows and you cut it, the new growth from the scalp will either be straight or wavy, depending on your natural hair type. On average, most people need treatment every 3–4 months. When your hair does not hold the style you desire and lacks body, it is then time to repeat the treatment.

Difference Between Salon and Home Treatments

A salon treatment differs from a home treatment primarily because most lotions used in salons contain chemicals that can damage hair when handled by inexperienced individuals, resulting in under-processing. Your stylist, however, has the technical knowledge and expertise to determine the ideal strength of solution for your hair and desired hairstyle. Moreover, their technical training and professional knowledge allow them to gauge the appropriate timing for each step.

Types of Treatment

Chemical hair treatments come in a variety of options, addressing the different needs of everyone, such as colouring, straightening, restructuring, etc.

Smoothening/Hair Relaxing

Smoothening is one of the oldest methods to tame curly hair. It is also the most cost-effective method. This treatment takes about three hours, depending on your hair texture, thickness, density, and length and lasts approximately for 4–5 months.

Hair Rebonding /Straightening

Rebonding is a chemical hair treatment that straightens the hair giving it some much-needed shine. Hair rebonding involves using a cream or relaxant to break the natural hair structure followed by a neutraliser to re-bond the hair structure. This treatment is ideal for those who have problems taming their thick or wavy hair. This process is performed according to the structure and thickness of your hair and could take about 5–8 hours.

It is usually on the expensive side but lasts longer than hair smoothening, approximately 6–12 months.

Keratin Treatment

Also known as 'Brazilian straightening', this treatment adds a coat of keratin to your hair, thereby replenishing its nutrients and making it soft, smooth, frizz-free, and straight. Keratin treatment can take about 1–4 hours, but it largely depends on the length and texture of your hair.

Hair Botox

It is a non-chemical, deep conditioning treatment that makes your hair smoother, shinier, and healthy-looking. It is an effective way to straighten your hair and make it less fussy. Hair Botox is the safest deep treatment as it does not contain formaldehyde or other harsh chemicals that end up weakening the hair.

Perm

Perm is an abbreviation of 'permanent wave'. It involves setting the hair into waves or curls using curling tools and lotions. One can opt for soft curls, wavy hair, tight curls, textured perms, spot perms, and much more. This treatment can last for a few months and, at times, even more than a year.

If you have decided to undergo a hair treatment, it is recommended to allocate 1.5 to 2.5 hours for the service. The most significant part of the treatment is the wrapping and straightening, which is also one of the most crucial aspects.

Thus, it is strongly advised not to rush your stylist during the process. Give them ample time to do their job properly. Additionally, if you are unsure of cutting your hair before or after the treatment, consult your professional stylist. Hair can be cut before the treatment as well, but it largely depends upon your stylist, your personal style preference, and the condition of your hair.

Choosing a Hairdresser

A good hairdresser is just as vital to pretty hair as the right hair-care equipment and the ideal style. However, a good hairdresser is hard to find. Here are some tips to help you in your search.

Your hairdresser should give you a style that fits both your hair type and your lifestyle. If you spend a great deal of time outdoors, on or off the job, you don't want a hairstyle that must be constantly protected from the weather elements. The same goes if you live in a damp or windy climate. Don't let anyone talk you into difficult hairstyles.

You must be able to manage your hair yourself between visits to the salon. Does your style look good only after it's been professionally done? Then, it may be time to find a new hairdresser who's a better stylist!

The cut should grow out gracefully, too. If it is scruffy and scraggy by the third week, the cut wasn't good to begin with. Even hair that grows rapidly should look good for about five to six weeks. One of the best ways to find a good hairdresser is through word of mouth – trial and error works, but the errors can be very trying. So, ask friends, neighbours, co-workers, and even strangers whose hairdos you like, for the name of their hairdresser. It's detective work that should pay off.

Proceeding with Care: Insights on Permanence

- There is no reason why anyone cannot undergo a chemical treatment; however, if you have abrasions on the skin or are dealing with an irritated scalp, it is advisable to tell your stylist and wait until the scalp issues are resolved before proceeding with the treatment.
- Some medications can accumulate on the hair shaft, which can impact the effectiveness of the treatment.
- Individuals who have damaged hair will need a series of treatments before undergoing any chemical treatment.
- Always consult your professional cosmetologist who can guide you through the proper procedures.

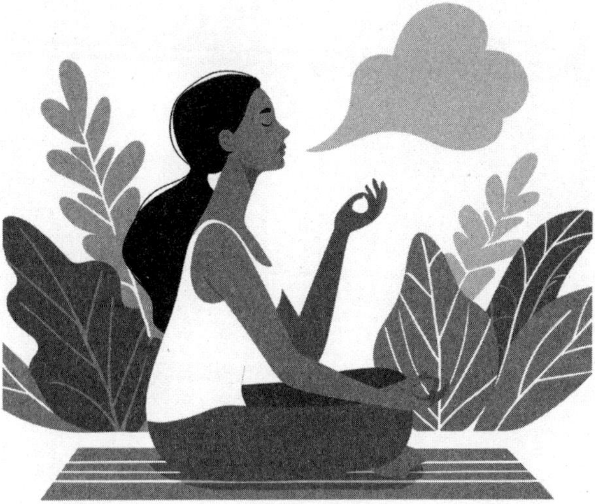

IV
BEAUTY FROM WITHIN

20
Exploring Your Food Choices

The word 'diet' conjures up visions of torture, hunger pangs, resisting temptations, and spending months on end trying to lose a few kilos, becoming more and more irritable as the months go by, and finding the bother not worth its while. But what if I told you that 'diet' really means having the cake and eating it, too? All you need is a simple plan.

Calories Needed To Maintain Your Desirable Weight
Daily Maintenance

	Age		
Desirable Weight in Pounds	**18–35**	**35–55**	**55–77**
99	1,700	1,500	1,300
110	1,850	1,650	1,400
121	2,000	1,750	1,550
128	2,100	1,900	1,600
132	2,150	1,950	1,650
143	2,300	2,050	1,800
154	2,400	2,150	1,850
165	2,550	2,300	1,950

When we consume more calories than necessary, these fatty substances are stored in our bodies and we accumulate more layers of fat, making us overweight.

What is a calorie? It is a measure of the amount of energy produced by food. Thus, foods high in calories make more energy. Energy generated is used by our bodies for walking, sitting and even sleeping. We gain weight when excess calories are taken.

Your Ideal Weight

It is important to keep in mind that weight can vary depending on age, bone structure, and genetic factors. To get an accurate measurement of your weight, it is recommended to measure yourself without clothes using a measuring tape. It is also useful to know that one pound of body weight is equivalent to 3,500 calories. The average adult consumes about 2,000 calories per day. To lose 2 pounds per week, one needs to follow a diet of 1,000 calories per day. Conversely, to gain 2 pounds per week, one needs to follow a diet of 3,000 calories per day. For those who are staying at home and not burning as much energy, a diet of 800 calories per day is necessary to lose 2 pounds per week.

Diet for Skin

Your skin is a true reflection of your inner health. Anything wrong inside is bound to show outside. A well-planned menu comprising a sensible and well-balanced diet ranks foremost in the skincare regime. To realise the impact of your diet on the skin, it is essential to be informed about what inadequacies and deficiencies in the diet can bring upon us.

Apart from diets to suit your individual needs and activities, there are basic principles of nutrition that apply to everyone—macronutrients that everyone must consume to live a healthy life, thereby maintaining that beautiful glow. Below is a general outline of a diet that can promote healthy skin:

1. Water: Drinking at least 8 glasses of water each day is crucial for keeping your skin hydrated and healthy. If you live in a hot climate or are active, you may need to drink even more.
2. Fruits and Vegetables: Eating a variety of colourful fruits and vegetables can provide your skin with vitamins, minerals, and antioxidants that aid in protecting it from damage. Consume more berries, citrus fruits, leafy greens, carrots, bell peppers, etc.
3. Healthy Fats: Omega-3 fatty acids found in foods like salmon, walnuts, and flaxseeds can help keep your skin hydrated and reduce inflammation.
4. Protein: It is essential for the repair and regeneration of skin. Include some lean sources of protein in your diet, such as fish, tofu, beans, and lentils.
5. Whole Grains: Whole grains like brown rice, quinoa, and oats provide vitamins, minerals, and fibre that support overall skin health.
6. Healthy Snacks: Instead of sugary or processed snacks, choose healthier options like nuts, seeds, yoghurt, or fresh fruit.
7. Consume Sugar and Processed Foods in Moderation: Diets high in sugar and processed foods can contribute to skin problems like acne and premature ageing. Go for whole, unprocessed foods instead.

8. Green Tea: Drinking green tea can improve skin health and protect against sun damage due to its high antioxidant content.
9. Probiotics: Foods rich in probiotics, such as yoghurt and kefir can help maintain a healthy balance of gut bacteria, which may, in turn, improve skin health.
10. Limit Alcohol and Caffeine: Consuming alcohol and caffeine in moderation and balancing them with plenty of water can prevent dehydration and keep your skin healthy.

Deficiency	Consequences
Vitamin A	• Thickening of skin texture • Wrinkles • Aggravation of acne
Vitamin B-complex	• Pale skin • Pigmentation • Dark circles under the eyes
Vitamin C	• Acne • Uneven skin tone
Vitamin E	• Pigmentation
Protein	• Loss of skin rejuvenation • Degeneration of the connective tissue underneath the skin surface
Minerals (zinc, calcium)	• Pale skin
Iron	• Pigmentation spots
Oil and Moisture	• Excessive skin dryness and chapping

Diet for Hair

A nutritious diet is essential for our growth, well-being, and longevity. The same is true for hair. Despite being the least important among human organs, hair receives minimal nutrition from the blood, which is left over after fulfilling the needs of vital organs, such as the heart, lungs, and liver. Consequently, hair often exhibits the first signs of nutritional deficiency in the body.

Hair is an extension of the skin, consisting of cells that have migrated from generative cells deeper within the body, formed four to six weeks earlier.

Given that hair is primarily composed of the protein called keratin, it needs adequate protein intake for optimal growth. Scientists have developed a method to assess the nutritional value of protein-rich foods, termed 'biological value', based on their ability to meet dietary needs.

Eggs contain the highest levels of the amino acid methionine among all complete proteins. Additionally, they are rich in vitamins A, B, D, and E, as well as minerals such as sulphur. One egg a day can significantly benefit your hair health.

Milk is not just for children, it's a complete source of protein with additional vitamins and minerals essential for healthy hair. Adults are advised to consume one glass of milk daily, along with a serving of paneer (cottage cheese) or yoghurt.

Yoghurt is a traditional health food, which is rich in lactic acid and nutrients that are easily absorbed by most individuals. It provides ample B-complex vitamins and beneficial bacteria, helping in digestion and overall well-being. Individuals taking antibiotics should consider consuming yoghurt daily to replenish the beneficial bacteria killed by the medication.

Sunflower seeds are low in calories and a rich source of complete protein, polyunsaturated fatty acids, vitamins, and minerals, making them an excellent addition to a hair-friendly diet.

While a balanced diet should ideally provide all the necessary nutrients, some individuals may benefit from vitamin supplements. However, excessive intake of fat-soluble vitamins (A, D, E, and K) can lead to liver damage. Water-soluble vitamins, such as those in the B-complex group, are safer as the body only absorbs what it needs. Vitamin B, crucial for healthy skin and hair, can also ease certain symptoms of premenstrual tension. Thus, a daily yeast tablet can prove to be beneficial. Yeast, resembling human body cells in composition, is a rich source of protein and vitamin B.

Hair enemies are often detrimental to overall health as well. When planning your diet, consider that many foods contain toxins or substances the body does not need or cannot utilise. These toxins must be eliminated, because they can burden your liver, kidneys, bowels, lungs, and sweat glands. Excessive toxin exposure may lead to various health issues, including hair and scalp problems such as reduced hair growth, excessive oiliness, or dandruff.

A diet high in snack foods, potato chips, cakes, pastries, white bread, high-carbohydrate foods, sugary soft drinks, factory-farmed meats, and vegetables may contain higher levels of toxins. While it may be challenging to avoid such foods entirely, minimising their consumption can contribute to overall health and hair well-being.

21

Move Your Body

It is widely recognised that exercise holds immense value for overall well-being. Not only does it help in toning muscles and shedding excess weight, but it also serves as an effective stress reliever, reducing the need for sleep aids and improving mood swings. Numerous medical experts advocate for regular exercise, particularly for women, as it can significantly reduce the risk of heart-related issues. Starting an exercise routine before reaching the age of 40 is strongly encouraged, as it can help maintain cardiovascular health and counterbalance the hormonal changes that occur during menopause. Additionally, consistent exercise promotes elasticity in blood vessels, improves circulation, and contributes to joint flexibility, which is particularly beneficial for those dealing with arthritis. Embracing a regular exercise regimen is often likened to a natural anti-ageing remedy, as it revitalises muscles, enhances tone and promotes overall agility.

Outdoor Exercises

If you are not fond of traditional exercise, outdoor sports can be an excellent alternative for you. However, don't rely solely on weekend sports activities to fulfil all your exercise needs. Even professional athletes need additional exercise to maintain fitness levels and improve their performance. You can engage in some of these outdoor activities:

a. Cycling: It is an excellent exercise for strengthening your lower body, particularly the muscles in the thighs, calves, and glutes. It's also a great cardiovascular workout, helping to improve heart health and stamina.
b. Walking and Jogging: Both walking and jogging can help strengthen and tone your muscles in the lower body. Regular walking or jogging can improve cardiovascular health, boost mood, and help you lose fat. Whether you prefer a brisk walk in nature or a heart-pumping jog through the city streets, incorporating these activities into your routine can help you tone your body and improve your overall health and fitness.
c. Ball Games: Games such as tennis, bowling, badminton, basketball, or squash act as good body stretchers. As these activities involve repeated arm motions, they can strengthen your upper body, while improving agility and quick reflexes, contributing to overall fitness.
d. Swimming: It is well-known for toning and strengthening the pectoral muscles that support the bust. It also tones the upper arms while fostering flexibility.

Everyday Exercises

As a working wife and mother, I understand the importance of exercises that are both easy and effective, allowing you to incorporate them into activities such as watching television, reading a magazine, talking on the phone, or playing cards.

Begin with five to ten-minute sessions and gradually increase their length as your body becomes accustomed to the conditioning.

You don't need special clothing to exercise; anything comfortable that allows freedom of movement will suffice. For floor routines, simply stretch out on your rug or carpet.

Whenever you engage in activities that involve bending, such as opening lower drawers of dressers or file cabinets, dusting furniture legs, or making beds, give your thigh muscles a workout by performing deep knee bends while keeping your back straight, bending your knees, and lowering your body onto your heels as you reach for the item you want.

Exercise your abdominal muscles while sewing, knitting, reading, or watching television by lifting one leg, straightening it parallel to the floor, and raising it as high as you can, then lowering it and repeating the movement with your other leg.

Reaching for items on the highest shelf or putting up curtains are also effective stretching exercises that can help strengthen your body and arms. As you reach up, tuck your bottom in, rise on your toes, and stretch all over.

All sweeping movements, such as with a broom, exercise your arm muscles. Make sure to use both your arms so that both sides are exercised equally.

Another exercise to tone your upper arms is to stretch out on your back in bed with your arms straight down at your sides. Spread your fingers and bend them slightly to form claws with the palms facing downwards. Press down with your hands as if you were trying to push your fingers right through the mattress, holding the pressure for a slow count of three, then relax. Repeat the exercise three times.

You can also exercise your abdominal muscles while on the telephone by bending forward from the hips and bouncing up and down, letting the hand that is not holding the telephone hang down. After a few bounces, straighten up, pull in your stomach, tighten your buttocks, and repeat. Then, bend to the side and see how far down your leg your hand can reach. Bounce sideways a few times and repeat the movement on the other side.

To tone your glute muscles, you can perform an exercise while engaging in sedentary activities such as watching TV, knitting, or reading. First, sit on a straight-backed hard chair with your back straight. Slowly lift your right leg, bending the knee, pointing your toes down, and lifting the leg as high as possible without causing strain. Hold for a while, then slowly return the leg to its original position. Repeat the exercise with your left leg, performing five repetitions with each leg.

To tone your thighs and bottom, try sitting on a hard chair both at home and at work. Practise tensing up your thigh muscles for a count of six at least 20 times a day.

While waiting for water to boil, exercise your calves and thighs by rising on your toes, then bending your knees until you are almost in a sitting position (while staying on your toes). Repeat this movement until the water boils.

It also is possible to exercise your body while playing card games such as bridge or rummy, even if you have a dowager's hump. To do this, you should sit in the correct position, pull up from your diaphragm, and hold the cards level with your eyes. As the cards are being dealt, toss your head as far back as you can and then drop your chin to your chest.

Even while taking a bath, you can engage in some stretching movements. Stand upright to wash your back and then reach down your back with one arm, then the other, while keeping your legs straight. Stretch from your waist to wash your ankles and toes. Between lathering, place the soap slightly out of reach so that you must stretch your arms to get it. Always remember to keep your core tight, as if you are trying to touch your stomach to your spine. This will help you strengthen your muscles in that area and flatten your stomach.

The significance of exercise for maintaining healthy and radiant skin cannot be overstated. Engaging in regular physical activity not only enhances blood circulation, delivering vital nutrients to the skin but also promotes the elimination of toxins, contributing to a clearer and healthier complexion. Furthermore, exercise aids in reducing stress levels, which can otherwise worsen skin conditions such as acne and eczema. By moving our body daily, we not only improve our overall health but also nurture the natural glow and vitality of our skin.

22
Unlocking Radiance through Massage

Self-massage has a rich history dating back to ancient civilisations, and its popularity continues to grow in modern times. With a diverse range of techniques and benefits, self-massage remains an accessible and effective method for relaxation, rejuvenation, and overall well-being. From ancient traditions to contemporary practices, the art of self-massage continues to be cherished and integrated into wellness routines worldwide.

Ayurveda in India

Ayurveda, an ancient Indian system of medicine, has a rich history of self-massage. Abhyanga, a traditional Ayurvedic self-massage technique, involves using warm herbal oils to massage the entire body, promoting relaxation, nourishment, and overall well-being.

Chinese Medicine

In Chinese medicine, self-massage techniques have been used for thousands of years. The practice of 'Qi Gong' includes self-massage to stimulate the flow of 'Qi' (vital energy) in the body and balance its energy channels (meridians).

Ancient Egypt

The ancient Egyptians were known for their beauty and wellness rituals, which included self-massage techniques using aromatic oils and natural ingredients. Massage was employed not solely for relaxation but also to promote skin health and maintain physical and spiritual balance.

Ancient Greece

In ancient Greece, massage was an integral part of the culture and was practised both professionally and personally. Greek athletes, for instance, used self-massage techniques to prepare their bodies for athletic competitions and recovery purposes.

Renaissance Era

During the Renaissance, self-massage became a popular practice among European aristocrats and the elite. They used fragrant oils and ointments to massage their bodies, believing it enhanced their beauty and helped maintain youthful skin.

Modern Times

In our modern, fast-paced world, carving out time for self-care is a challenge. However, there is one self-care practice that can easily be incorporated into your routine—head-to-toe self-massage. Beyond just a luxurious indulgence, this holistic approach to relaxation offers numerous benefits for both the body and mind. Below are some advantages of head-to-toe self-massage, the techniques involved, and the transformative effects it can have on your well-being.

Benefits of Head-to-Toe Self-Massage

1. Stress Relief: Head-to-toe self-massage is a potent stress buster. As you knead and massage your muscles, the body releases endorphins—natural mood elevators—promoting a sense of relaxation and contentment.
2. Improved Circulation: The gentle pressure and strokes during self-massage stimulate blood flow throughout the body. Improved circulation ensures that essential nutrients and oxygen reach all cells and tissues while facilitating the removal of metabolic waste.
3. Muscle Tension Reduction: Self-massage targets areas of muscle tension, tightness, and soreness, releasing knots and promoting muscle flexibility.
4. Pain Management: For those experiencing minor aches and pains, self-massage can be highly therapeutic. The manipulation of soft tissues can provide relief from discomfort as well as promote healing.
5. Mental Calmness: Engaging in head-to-toe self-massage is akin to a meditative practice. It encourages mindfulness and brings focus to the present moment, leading to reduced mental chatter and increased calmness.
6. Enhanced Sleep Quality: By incorporating self-massage into your bedtime routine, you signal your body to unwind, creating a peaceful transition to sleep and potentially reducing sleep disturbances.
7. Skin Nourishment: Using natural oils or lotions during self-massage can improve skin health by

enhancing moisture retention, promoting elasticity, and imparting a radiant glow.

8. Detoxification Support: Certain self-massage techniques, such as lymphatic drainage, can aid in the removal of toxins, supporting the body's natural detoxification processes.
9. Emotional Well-Being: Head-to-toe self-massage boosts self-awareness and self-compassion. This practice allows you to tune into your emotions, reducing symptoms of anxiety and depression.
10. Boosted Immune System: Regular self-massage helps stimulate the lymphatic system, which plays an important role in supporting the immune system's function.
11. Improved Posture: By addressing areas like the neck and shoulders, self-massage can alleviate tension and discomfort associated with poor posture, encouraging better alignment.
12. Empowerment and Independence: Embracing head-to-toe self-massage empowers individuals to take charge of their well-being, promoting self-sufficiency in maintaining health.
13. Accessible Self-Care: Unlike professional massages, self-massage is accessible to everyone. It can be practised at any time, in any space, and without additional expenses.
14. A Ritual of Self-Love: Incorporating head-to-toe self-massage into your routine is an act of self-love and self-nurturing, reinforcing the importance of honouring your body and mind.

Head Massage

A scalp massage has the potential to induce a calming effect on the nerves, stimulate glandular secretions, and enhance the circulation of blood and lymphatic fluids. Head massage not only stimulates hair growth but also helps prevent hair loss.

Within the domain of massage therapy, there exist techniques that possess the power to elevate the effectiveness of treatments through skilful scalp manipulation. Moreover, these techniques extend their influence on the face and neck, stimulating rejuvenation. As hands glide across these regions, a remarkable transformation unfolds—a gentle stimulation of blood circulation follows, caressing the scalp and neck while simultaneously soothing the delicate nerves that reside within the depths of the mind. Such is the potency of these techniques that individuals are transported into a state of blissful tranquillity, instantaneously immersed in a realm of deep relaxation.

The correct way for a head massage is to stimulate the scalp by using your fingertips and the cushion of your palms. Use gentle, circular motions, rhythmically massaging the scalp and hair for enhanced relaxation.

Hairline

Position your fingertips at the hairline, extending towards the top of your ears. Curve your palms and apply gentle pressure with your fingers on the scalp. Begin moving your fingers in circular motions, massaging along the hairline while focusing on areas affected by hair loss. Continue the massage, enclosing the temples, the area behind the ears, and the back of your neck.

Forehead

Steady your neck by placing your left hand across the back of your head. Allow your head to relax on your hand while positioning your right hand across your forehead. Extend your thumb and forefingers across your brow line, moving your hand slowly and firmly up to one inch beyond your hairline.

Scalp Manipulation

- Place your palms firmly against the scalp above the ears and perform circular movements, lifting and lowering the scalp.
- Repeat the circular motion with one hand at the top front of the head and the other at the nape.
- Position your fingertips on the sides of the head and gently slide them upwards, spreading your fingers as you move towards the top of your head. Gently massage in a circular motion, then slowly move your fingers outwards and towards the back.
- Place your left hand across your forehead and use the fingertips of your right hand to give a gentle circular massage at the base of the skull, moving from the left ear to the right ear.
- Using your fingertips, perform firm up-and-down motions from side to side, starting from the crown and moving towards the hairline. Reverse the direction and repeat.
- Hold small bunches of hair gently with your fingertips and pull slowly for a count of eight, then release.

Repeat this process, tugging the hair throughout the entire head.

Different Modes of Massage

Massaging the scalp properly can offer various benefits. Here are the different modes of massaging your scalp.

1. Circles at the Side of Your Head: Gently position your fingers on the scalp, approximately one inch above the ear, using one hand at a time. Remember to keep the other hand in place to sustain uninterrupted contact throughout the process.
2. Circles behind the Ears to the Top of the Head: Raise one hand consecutively, starting with either hand and position your fingers approximately one inch behind the ears. Gently touching the scalp.
3. Back of the Head: Place both hands together, forming a cup-like shape, and position them on the top of your head, specifically on the bone structure. Utilising the heels of your hands, perform three rotations at the crown area. Then, lift each hand individually and relocate them to the middle back of your head. Proceed to execute three circular movements in this region.
4. Nape: Raise your hands individually and carefully position them on the nape of your neck. Then, proceed to perform three rotations in that area.
5. Rotating the Nape: Hold your forehead with one hand, securing a firm grasp. On the other hand, form a cupping shape and position it on the right side of the back of your head, on the crest of the occipital bone.

Place the heel of your hand in the hollow region of the nape, directly beneath the bone. Proceed to rotate your hands three times, alternating between left and right movements. Repeat all movements five times each.

Neck Massage

A neck massage offers numerous benefits, including the release of accumulated tension in the area, acting as a beauty treatment, cleansing and conditioning the skin, and improving blood circulation. To enhance its effectiveness, using oil or moisturiser can be beneficial, as the skin absorbs the product during the massage, further promoting blood circulation. While existing lines may not be removed, this practice can help prevent the development of new lines.

The four primary movements of a neck massage are as follows:

- Stroking—induces a calming effect
- Kneading—stimulates the neck muscles
- Pressure—prompts the neck muscles
- Gentle slapping—also stimulates the neck muscles

It is important to note that an effective neck massage exerts slight pressure using firm yet gentle movements.

Steps to Massage Your Neck

First, take some moisturiser. To target the front of your neck, begin by using one hand and then the other to perform gentle strokes from the chin down to the cleavage, extending towards the armpit area. This technique assists in the proper drainage of lymphatic fluid. Ensure that the movements are both deep and swift for optimal results.

Gently place one hand on the collarbone. Then, using three fingers, softly stroke from the base of your throat, moving upwards along the neck towards the chin, and finally, continue the stroke outwards to the edge of the jaw, reaching the earlobe. It is crucial to keep the strokes extremely light, resembling the delicate touch of a feather.

Using your thumb and forefinger, pinch the skin along your jawbone, gradually moving from the chin towards the earlobe.

Make rapid stroking movements with your fingers, using the back of your hands, beginning from the neck's base, and moving upwards and outwards from beneath your chin.

For the final stage of the neck massage on the front, employ gentle slapping motions from the collarbone upwards along the neck, moving towards the chin. Utilise your fingers on the neck and the back of your hand beneath the chin. This technique can stimulate the neck muscles and enhance blood circulation.

Gently massaging the back of your neck can help alleviate built-up stress and relieve pain. To do this, follow these steps:

1. Position your hands to cup the contours of your neck. Place one hand at the bottom of the neck and the other at the base of the skull.
2. Apply light pressure as you pull each hand gently in opposite directions. Make sure not to use excessive force to avoid damaging collagen.

3. Rotate your fingers in a circular motion, gradually moving from the base of your neck toward the shoulders.

Remember, all the movements should be performed with a light touch to prevent any potential collagen breakage.

Face Massage

Massage is an essential part of skincare. It keeps the face muscles toned and firm, thereby preventing sagging of the skin. When applying moisturiser in the morning or at night, take a little extra time to turn your beauty routine into a therapeutic massage treatment that will make you feel good, both mentally and physically.

Massage helps keep skin pores healthy and increases the action of the excretory glands, helping your skin to cleanse itself. Massage arouses tissues, perks up every little cell, and creates a tingling feeling of well-being while improving circulation.

A correct massage technique relieves nervous tension and eases out the fine lines. It also strengthens face and throat muscles and removes scaly, dead skin, leaving it smooth, firm, and glowing.

Most muscles flow in a general upward and outward direction, which is why you should apply most face creams in this manner. It is important to massage in the direction that the muscles flow, as incorrect movements can pull muscles and cause them to sag. Be particularly careful to use a delicate movement near the eyes, where it is easy to stretch the skin and cause bagginess.

How to Massage

- Using plenty of cream, start at the base of your throat, massaging from the collarbone to the tip of the chin and jaws. wherein one hand follows the other in deep stroking movements. Repeat each movement 10 times.
- Using your index finger and thumb, pinch or stroke from your chin to the ends of your jawbone and back several times.
- Gently slap the skin under your chin with the back of your hands. This helps with boosting circulation.
- Move on to treat your cheek muscles by working from your chin up across your cheeks to your temples with an upwards and outwards circling movement of your fingertips.
- Puff out your cheeks. Pat with fingertips along the laugh line, from the corners of the mouth up to the nose. Massage your nose with small, circular movements, from the bridge of your nose to the nose tip.
- Massage under the eyes, from outer to inner corners and over the eyelids. Using the second and third fingers, sweep lightly out around your eyes in a gentle, stroking movement from the bridge of your nose around to your temples, following the bone of your eyes.
- With quick little taps of your fingertips, as if playing a piano, move from the inner corners to the outer corners of your eyes, concentrating on the little crow's feet.

- To relieve tension, pinch your eyebrows, working from the bridge of your nose outwards, and make small circles at the temples.
- Use a brisk scissor movement of your first and second fingers and dance the fingertips horizontally up and over your forehead. Begin at the centre of your forehead and finish at your temples. Then, stroke up between your eyes and over your forehead using your ring and middle fingers, and finish at your temples.
- There are two pressure points, one at the bridge of your nose where it meets your eye socket, and the other at your temple just level with the ends of your eyebrow. Gentle pressure applied at these points with your fingertips and maintained for five seconds can be relaxing.
- Massage for about 5–10 minutes daily or 20 minutes once a week.

Body Massage

In our quest for holistic well-being, self-body massage stands as a timeless practice that brings harmony to the body and mind. Beyond being a luxurious indulgence, self-massage offers several benefits, including relaxation, stress relief, and improved circulation. In this comprehensive guide, we will explore different massage strokes that can be used for a self-body massage and delve into step-by-step instructions on how to massage different body parts, allowing you to embark on a journey of self-care and rejuvenation.

Tools for Self-Body Massage

1. Massage Oil or Cream: Choose a high-quality massage oil or cream that suits your skin type. Options like coconut oil, almond oil, or jojoba oil work well for most people.
2. Massage Tools: While your hands are enough for many areas, consider investing in massage tools like a foam roller, massage balls, or a wooden massager for hard-to-reach spots or deeper pressure.
3. Comfortable Space: Create a serene ambience by dimming the lights, playing soft music, and ensuring the room temperature is comfortable.

Massage Strokes

1. Effleurage: Originating from the French, meaning, 'to skim', this gentle and gliding stroking movement involves using flat palms to apply long, flowing movements along the body. Effleurage is ideal for warming up the muscles, spreading massage oil or lotion, and inducing relaxation.
2. Petrissage: It entails kneading, squeezing, and lifting the skin and underlying tissues. By applying firm pressure, this technique helps release muscle tension and increase blood flow.
3. Friction: It involves using circular motions with the fingertips or thumbs to apply pressure to specific points. This stroke is perfect for targeting knots and adhesions, promoting the release of muscle tension.

4. Tapotement: It consists of rhythmic tapping, patting, or hacking movements. It invigorates the muscles, enhances circulation, and provides a stimulating effect.
5. Vibration: Vibration includes gentle shaking or trembling movements, which can help in relaxing the muscles and promoting a sense of calm.

Self-Body Massage Techniques for Different Body Parts

Step 1: Preparing for the Massage

Create a calm ambience by dimming the lights, playing soothing music, and ensuring that your space is comfortable and free from distractions. Start with a few deep breaths to centre yourself.

Step 2: Neck and Shoulders

- Begin with effleurage strokes on your neck and shoulders, using both hands to massage in a circular motion. Gradually apply more pressure to warm up the muscles and encourage relaxation.
- Move on to the petrissage technique, gently squeezing and lifting the muscles. Focus on areas of tension, such as the upper trapezius, and knead in a circular motion.
- Use friction on specific knots or tight spots, applying firm pressure with your fingertips or thumbs. Allow the tension to release as you work through these areas.
- Conclude with tapotement, lightly tapping or patting the neck and shoulders to invigorate and stimulate blood flow.

Step 3: Arms and Hands

- Apply massage oil or lotion to your arms and hands, using the effleurage motion to spread it evenly and warm up the muscles.
- Use petrissage to knead and gently pull the muscles, paying attention to the biceps, triceps, and forearm muscles.
- Apply friction to the forearms and palms, focusing on any tense areas and using circular motions to release tension.
- Finish with tapotement, lightly tapping or hacking along the arms and gently patting the hands to awaken and refresh.

Step 4: Back

- Start by using a foam roller or massage balls on your back to target any knots or tight areas.
- Begin effleurage strokes along your spine, working your way outwards, to the sides of your back. Use both hands to create a soothing, flowing motion.
- Employ petrissage on either side of the spine, gently kneading and lifting the muscles to release tension.
- Apply friction to areas with knots or tightness, using circular motions to encourage the release of muscle adhesions.
- Conclude with tapotement, lightly tapping or hacking along the back to invigorate and awaken the senses.

Step 5: Legs and Feet

- Massage your legs from the thighs to the calves, using effleurage to warm up the muscles and spread the oil.
- Move on to petrissage, kneading and gently pulling your thigh and calf muscles. Focus on any tight spots and use circular motions to release tension.
- Apply friction to the quadriceps and calves, especially targeting areas with knots or soreness.
- Finish with tapotement, lightly tapping along the legs to increase circulation and promote a sense of vitality.
- Pay extra attention to your feet, using your thumbs to apply pressure and circular motions to the soles. Massage each toe individually, applying gentle pressure.

Lymphatic Drainage Massage

Lymphatic drainage massage involves stimulating the lymphatic system, which plays a vital role in the body's immune function by clearing out waste, toxins, and excess fluids from tissues. By employing gentle, rhythmic movements, this massage method assists in transporting lymph fluid throughout the body, facilitating its passage through lymph nodes for eventual elimination.

Lymphatic drainage massage aims to optimise lymphatic system function, promote detoxification, reduce swelling and inflammation, support immune function, and contribute to a heightened sense of relaxation and well-being.

This massage helps those undergoing detoxification as it removes toxins from thc body as well as in overall wellness and relaxation. It can also be used post-surgery to reduce swelling and expedite the healing process. Those suffering from Lymphedema can also opt for this massage as it aids in managing swelling.

How to Massage

You can perform some self-massage techniques at home to help stimulate lymphatic flow. Here are some general guidelines for self-lymphatic drainage massage:

- Remember to breathe deeply throughout the process of lymphatic stimulation
- Drink enough water
- Remember to not apply excess pressure

Steps:

1. Start by placing your fingers around your clavicle or collarbone and gently make 5–8 circles at the base of your neck on both sides.
2. Move your fingers to the area right below your ears and make small circles along the sides of your neck.
3. Now focus on your armpits, making 5–10 circles in each. Similarly, target the groin, again making 5–10 circles.
4. Next, place your hands right under your ribcage, with part of the hand on the ribcage and part below it. With your fingers facing upwards, move your palms to drain the area.
5. Find the crease of your groin and massage this area in a circular motion.

6. Then go to the back of your knees and gently pump the hollow of this area a few times.
7. End the massage by making small circles on both sides of your ankles.

Incorporate these techniques into your daily routine to promote lymphatic drainage and ensure overall well-being.

Professional Massages and How to Choose

Professional body massages come in various types, each with its unique techniques and benefits. Here are some common types of body massages offered by professionals, along with tips on how to choose the right one for you.

Swedish Massage

This is one of the most popular and widely practised massages worldwide. It uses a combination of long, gliding strokes, kneading, friction, tapping, and gentle stretching.

Best for: Relaxation, stress relief, muscle tension, and overall well-being.

Deep Tissue Massage

Focuses on targeting deeper layers of muscles and connective tissue. Uses slow, firm pressure and techniques to release chronic muscle tension and knots.

Best for: Chronic pain, muscle tightness, sports-related injuries, and improving flexibility.

Hot Stone Massage

This involves placing heated smooth stones on specific points of the body and using them to massage. The warmth of the stones helps relax muscles and promotes circulation.

Best for: Relaxation, muscle tension, and improving blood flow.

Aromatherapy Massage

It incorporates essential oils, which are chosen for their specific therapeutic properties. The massage techniques used are often like Swedish massage.

Best for: Relaxation, stress relief, mood enhancement, and overall well-being.

Thai Massage

This is an ancient form of massage that involves stretching and applying gentle pressure along the energy lines of the body. The recipient remains clothed during the massage, and no oils are used.

Best for: Improving flexibility, energy flow, and reducing muscle tension.

Sports Massage

It is geared towards athletes and active individuals and combines various techniques to help prevent injuries, improve performance, and aid in recovery.

Best for: Athletes, sports enthusiasts, and those who perform heavy physical activities.

Shiatsu Massage

It originated in Japan and involved applying pressure with fingers, thumbs, and palms to specific points on the body. The goal is to stimulate the body's energy flow.

Best for: Balancing energy, reducing stress, and promoting relaxation.

Prenatal Massage

This massage is designed for expectant mothers to help alleviate pregnancy-related discomforts. Uses specialised positioning and techniques to ensure the safety and comfort of both the mother and baby.

Best for: Relieving pregnancy discomforts, reducing stress, and promoting relaxation.

How to Choose the Right Massage

1. Identify Your Goals: Consider your specific needs and what you want to achieve with the massage—relaxation, pain relief, or improved flexibility. Different massages cater to various goals.
2. Consult with a Professional: If you're unsure which massage is best for you, consult with a licensed massage therapist. They can assess your individual needs and recommend the most suitable massage.
3. Consider Your Preferences: Think about your comfort level with pressure, oils, and other factors. For instance, if you prefer gentle pressure and aromatherapy, a Swedish or Aromatherapy massage might be a good fit.
4. Check for Specialised Massages: If you have specific conditions or preferences, look for specialised massages like prenatal massage for expectant mothers or reflexology for foot-focused therapy.

5. Communicate with the Therapist: Communicate your preferences, any health concerns, or areas of focus with the massage therapist before the session begins. A good therapist will customise the massage to meet your needs.
6. Try Different Types: Don't be afraid to explore different types of massages to find the one that resonates with you the most. Each massage offers unique benefits, and you may discover a favourite.

Self-massage is a simple yet powerful practice that offers myriad benefits for both the body and mind. By using the above-mentioned techniques, you can easily alleviate muscle tension, improve circulation, and promote relaxation.

23
INNER BEAUTY

I have always practised and preached that beauty is holistic; it is not just skin deep. Our outer beauty reflects our inner beauty. This quest for holistic beauty led me to study numerous alternative therapies and I went on to learn and practise reiki, pranic healing, Arhatic Yoga, crystal therapy, colour therapy, NLP, and much more.

I am also a trained happiness and mindfulness coach and have experienced and witnessed the tremendous impact that emotions have over not only your wellness but also your skin and hair. They play a key role in one's wellness and beauty. Emotions help to uplift or reduce your vibrations and energy. We vibrate at certain levels, and that determines our happiness or sadness.

If you are feeling depressed, sad, angry, grieving, or sick, your vibration is low. It also reflects on the physical level. To elevate your state, you will need to raise your vibrations to happiness, peace, and compassion.

Beauty Blockers

Let us talk about some emotions that act as beauty blockers. These emotions are so strong that they show on one's face. Anger, sadness, stress, worry, and fear are some of the emotions that manifest as wellness and skin or hair issues.

Anger

It is like a storm in your wellness landscape. Chronic anger can bring on a torrent of health issues, from heart problems and high blood pressure to weakened immunity. Let's not forget about the toll it takes on your mental health. Anxiety, depression, and strained relationships can be part of this deal.

When anger flares up, it sets off a chain reaction in your body, including the release of cortisol, the stress hormone. This can lead to oily skin, causing pesky breakouts. Furthermore, constant frowning due to anger can speed up the ageing process, resulting in premature fine lines. Even your hair may not escape the impact, as conditions like hair shedding become more noticeable during prolonged periods of anger.

Fear

Fear can cast a shadow over your wellness landscape, affecting your heart health, immune function, and mental well-being. Prolonged or excessive fear can kick-start the fight-or-flight response, leading to a rise in stress hormones and leaving you on the edge for a longer period.

When fear sets in, stress hormones go berserk, often resulting in skin reactions like hives, rashes, or allergic flare-ups. Dry skin and pigmentation are also results of fear. The fear-induced stress can trigger temporary hair thinning or loss, making it a double whammy for your appearance.

Worry

Worrying too much is akin to having a pesky mosquito buzzing around your wellness space. Chronic worry heightens anxiety and stress levels, disrupting sleep patterns, weakening your immune system, and causing a mental fog that's hard to shake off. It can even take its toll on your overall cognitive function.

Worrying often leads to increased cortisol levels, which can wreak havoc on your skin. It's like an open invitation for acne to make an appearance, and if you're already dealing with skin conditions like eczema or psoriasis, worry can escalate these issues. As for your hair, excessive worry can make your hair fall worse and increase oiliness and dandruff, making you worry even more!

Beauty Enhancers

Emotional beauty enhancers focus on nurturing inner well-being, boosting positive emotions, and cultivating a sense of contentment and fulfilment. These beauty enhancers play a vital role in your overall well-being.

Happiness

Happiness is your inner glow where you feel good, and your vibrations are high. It makes you want to get up and do things. Happiness must be cultivated every time; however, it does not stay with you all the time. Here is how you can hack happiness chemicals.

Dopamine

Often referred to as the 'feel-good' neurotransmitter, dopamine is associated with pleasure, reward, and motivation. To stimulate dopamine production, you can:

- Engage in physical exercise and activities you enjoy
- Set and achieve small, attainable goals
- Listen to your favourite music
- Try new experiences and adventures
- Rewarding yourself once you achieve anything

Endorphins

Endorphins act as natural painkillers and mood enhancers, providing feelings of euphoria while reducing stress. Here are some activities that can help to stimulate endorphin production:

- Engage in vigorous exercise, such as running, dancing, or high-intensity workouts
- Laughter and humour, such as watching a comedy show or spending time with friends
- Eat dark chocolate or spicy foods in moderation
- Practise deep breathing and relaxation exercises

Oxytocin

Oxytocin is often referred to as the 'love hormone' or 'bonding hormone' because it's associated with social bonding, trust, and empathy. Some activities to stimulate oxytocin production:

- Hug a loved one or cuddle with a pet
- Engage in positive social interactions and spend time with friends and family
- Practice acts of kindness and generosity towards others

- Participate in group activities and team sports

Serotonin

Serotonin is essential for regulating mood, sleep, appetite, and social behaviour. Low levels of serotonin are linked to depression and anxiety. To stimulate serotonin production, do these activities:

- Exposure to sunlight and spending time outdoors
- Regular exercise, especially aerobic activities
- Engage in acts of kindness and contribute to your community
- Practice meditation and relaxation techniques

One way to experience happiness is by smiling. Have you heard the popular saying: 'Smile and the world smiles with you'? A smile spreads happiness. Did you know that an average adult smiles 20 times a day and a child smiles 400 times a day? Every time you smile, each cell of your body unconsciously feels everything is all right. We have trillions of cells inside us, and we can light them up with happiness just by smiling.

Smiling plays a significant role in inducing happiness and is often considered a universal expression of joy, positivity, and friendliness. The act of smiling, whether genuine or even a deliberate, intentional smile, can have a significant impact on our emotions and overall well-being.

In all my years as a happiness coach, I tell people how important it is for your smile to reach your eyes. When you are happy, your eyes smile. The best way to do it is to think of a happy moment in your life and then smile; it will always reach your eyes.

Here's how smiling contributes to inducing happiness:

1. Induces Neurotransmitters: Smiling triggers the release of neurotransmitters, such as endorphins, serotonin, and dopamine in the brain.
2. Reduces Stress and Anxiety: Smiling, even in challenging situations, can reduce stress by decreasing cortisol levels, a hormone associated with stress.
3. Boosts the Immune System: Smiling has been linked to a strong immune system. The release of endorphins and other positive chemicals can support your immune function, helping you stay healthier and more resilient against illnesses.
4. Enhances Social Interaction and Connection: Smiling is a powerful social cue that signals approachability, openness, and friendliness. Smiling comes easily to me and I have seen that when I smile at others, it leads to better social interactions.
5. Elevates Mood and Well-Being: The physical act of smiling, regardless of its origin, can send signals to your brain, encouraging it to adopt a positive emotional state. This can lift your mood and overall sense of well-being, providing a natural and accessible way to generate happiness.
6. Spreads Happiness: Smiling is contagious. When you smile at someone, they are likely to smile back, creating a ripple effect of positivity. Sharing smiles with others can create a more joyful and harmonious

environment, improving the happiness of those around you.

7. Improves Self-Perception: Smiling can positively impact how you perceive yourself. When you smile, you convey self-assuredness, confidence, and happiness, which can boost your self-esteem and self-image.

Gratitude

Gratitude is like an elixir for the soul that unlocks a host of benefits for our overall wellness. When we embrace gratitude, we invite a shift in perspective—an opportunity to focus on the positive aspects of our lives, no matter how big or small. I have been practising gratitude for a long time now. When things don't happen the way I want them to, when I am not reaching my goals, I pause to think that it is happening to me now because something better is going to come my way.

I once had an interesting encounter with a woman who had lost her business. When she asked me for advice, I suggested that, perhaps, she needed to change her direction, which might have been why she lost her business. A year later, I met her again, and to my delight, she had transitioned into a new field and was thriving far more than she had in the five years of her previous venture. Thus, if we practise gratitude for whatever is happening to us, then our mindset changes and better things come our way.

It is essential to express gratitude not just to people but to things, birds, animals, nature, and more. You can express gratitude without words and for no reason. Gratitude is not about others; it is about us feeling good.

It is a good idea to start your day with gratitude. Say, if you are going for a morning walk, you can feel immense gratitude for being able to experience all the good things around you. You can also feel gratitude for your house help in doing your chores. These are some small ways in which you can practise and express gratitude.

I once heard of this story of a bird in a desert. One day an angel was passing by the desert on his way to visit God. He saw this miserable bird without feathers, nearly dying.

He stopped to ask the bird, 'What happened to you?'

The bird asked the angel where he was going. The angel told him he was going to visit God.

The bird said, 'Please ask God to do something for me. I am so miserable. There is no food here. I have no feathers. It is so hot, and I am nearly dying. Please tell God to get me out of this misery.'

The angel asked God about the bird and if he could do something. God sent a message to the bird, through the angel, to feel gratitude for all that was happening. The bird agreed. The angel went on his way after conveying the message.

Six months later, the angel was crossing the same desert to meet God. To his surprise, he saw that the bird was hale and hearty, full of colourful feathers, singing beautiful tunes. He asked the bird how this miracle had occurred.

The bird said, 'I just did what God asked me to do. I felt grateful for all that was happening and soon everything started to change for me.'

This is the power of gratitude.

Benefits of Practising Gratitude

1. Enhanced Mental Health: Gratitude acts as a soothing balm for a restless mind. By acknowledging the good

in our lives, we reduce stress, anxiety, and depression. Gratitude provides us with a fresh perspective to view challenges, helping us develop resilience and a positive outlook.

2. Improved Physical Health: The ripple effect of gratitude doesn't stop at the mind; it extends to the body. Studies suggest that practising gratitude can lead to lower blood pressure, better immune function, and improved sleep. A grateful heart nurtures a healthier body.
3. Strengthened Relationships: Expressing gratitude nurtures and strengthens our relationships. When we share our appreciation for others, it deepens connections and promotes a culture of kindness and understanding. Gratitude builds bridges that connect hearts.
4. Heightened Sense of Happiness: Gratitude is a direct route to joy. When we take time to reflect on what we're thankful for, we cultivate a sense of contentment and happiness. It's like having a treasure map to your well of joy!
5. Increased Resilience: Life's challenges can be tough, but gratitude provides us with a shield of resilience, which helps us bounce back from adversity, find lessons in difficulties, and embrace growth through even the toughest of times.

Easy and Heartfelt Gratitude Practices

Now that we understand the magic that gratitude weaves into our lives, let's explore some simple and heartfelt ways to incorporate gratitude into our daily routine:

1. Gratitude Journalling: Start a gratitude journal where you jot down three things you're thankful for each day. These can range from a smile from a stranger to a beautiful sunset. Let your heart's whispers fill the pages. I usually end the day by writing down three or five things that I feel gratitude towards. It helps me to look at the good that happened during the day, and it often helps me realise that the day was not as bad as I thought it to be. It could also be a morning practice.
2. Gratitude Walks: During your walks, immerse yourself in gratitude. Observe the beauty of nature around you and silently express thanks for the vibrant world that surrounds you.
3. Gratitude Jar: Place a jar in your home and encourage family members to jot down things they're grateful for and drop them in. Read these notes together periodically for a heart-warming reminder of life's blessings.
4. Gratitude for Challenges: When faced with a challenge, take a moment to thank it for the lessons it brings. Challenges are often our greatest teachers, helping us grow stronger and wiser.
5. Gratitude Letters: Write a heartfelt letter to someone you're grateful for and share how they've positively impacted your life. You can choose to send it or simply keep it as a cherished reminder of gratitude.

Forgiveness

I cannot emphasise enough how forgiveness guides us towards a life of joy and contentment. When we hold a grudge against someone about something they have said or done, and harbour anger towards people or situations, we are only harming ourselves. Only forgiveness can liberate us from these feelings.

Forgiveness frees us from emotional shackles. It allows us to release anger, pain, and grudges, offering a sense of liberation and emotional freedom that can feel like a weight lifted off our shoulders. There are multiple other reasons to forgive:

- Emotional Harmony: Forgiveness leads to emotional equilibrium, providing a stable foundation for happiness and serenity in our daily lives.
- Healthy Relationships: In nurturing an environment of forgiveness, our relationships flourish.
- Positive Outlook: Forgiveness is an essential ingredient for maintaining a positive outlook on life. It allows us to see the good in ourselves, in others, and the world around us.
- Fosters inner growth: Forgiveness catalyses personal growth and transformation. It challenges us to rise above negative experiences, learn valuable life lessons, and evolve into better versions of ourselves.

Forgiveness is not for others but for us. There are so many instances in life when we make mistakes, but we simply go through with them. This leads to feelings of guilt, reduced self-confidence, and being miserable, blaming ourselves and not forgiving ourselves.

To illustrate what I am saying, let us look at a situation when two friends in a car met with a terrible accident. The passenger gets injured very seriously, and the driver miraculously escapes with minor injuries. The friend driving the car blames himself for what happened, although the accident occurred due to a truck that suddenly appeared from a side lane. But he could not forgive himself and went into alcohol abuse since he could not deal with what had happened to his friend. It was only after several counselling sessions that the person started to deal with this issue.

He wrote a letter to himself stating, 'I am aware of all that went wrong. And I know I could have done better. I take complete responsibility for all that I have done.' He then listed all the things that he felt guilty about, folded the paper, and wrote on top, 'I forgive myself,' in big letters. He burnt this letter, had a tall glass of water, and observed how the water soothed and forgave him.

This exercise will work for everyone. You can do this every few days, every month, or whenever you feel the need. This will help us to get on with life.

Here are a few simple forgiveness hacks:

1. Self-Reflection and Acceptance: Begin by reflecting on past actions and experiences. Acknowledge mistakes without self-judgment, understanding that they do not define you. Accept yourself with love and kindness, paving the way for self-forgiveness.
2. Gratitude for Lessons Learnt: Express gratitude for the lessons learnt from past actions or situations. Recognise that these experiences, although challenging, have contributed to your growth and wisdom.

3. The Power of Compassion: Cultivate compassion towards yourself and others. Understand that everyone is navigating their unique journey, with flaws and imperfections. Approach yourself and others with empathy and understanding.
4. Mindfulness and Letting Go: Practice mindfulness to stay present and cultivate a forgiving attitude. When negative thoughts arise, acknowledge them, and consciously choose to let them go, allowing space for forgiveness to enter.
5. Expressing Feelings: Find healthy ways to express your feelings, through journalling or talking to a trusted friend or therapist. Venting and releasing pent-up emotions can also be crucial towards forgiveness.

Forgiveness is a transformative practice that holds the key to unlocking our true potential for happiness and fulfilment.

Mindfulness

Mindfulness is quite a buzzword across the globe and leaders of all kinds—financial, political, and social—are seen talking about how it has played a vital role in their success story. Mindfulness is a gentle practice that has the incredible power to bring peace, clarity, and happiness into our daily lives.

It is a state of being fully present in the moment, paying attention to what's happening both inside and outside of ourselves without judgment. It's about being aware of our thoughts, emotions, and surroundings without getting caught up in them.

Benefits of Mindfulness

1. Reduced Stress: Mindfulness offers calmness in our busy lives, reducing stress and providing a sense of relaxation.
2. Enhanced Focus and Concentration: By training our minds to be present, we sharpen our focus, improving productivity and efficiency in daily tasks.
3. Improved Mental Health: Practicing mindfulness regularly can alleviate anxiety, depression, and other mental health challenges, promoting a more positive outlook on life.
4. Emotional Resilience: Mindfulness equips us with the tools to respond to challenging situations with a clear and composed mind, boosting emotional resilience.
5. Deeper Relationships: Being fully present with others cultivates deep connections and empathy, enhancing our relationships and fostering a sense of community.

Mindfulness Exercises

Here are some easy mindfulness exercises to kick-start your journey. Start with everyday acts like eating, walking, and working and slowly build them up:

Mindful Eating

- Choose a snack or a small meal
- Before taking a bite, notice the colours, textures, and aromas of the food
- Take a bite and savour the flavours and the sensation of chewing

Be fully present with each bite, appreciating the nourishment it provides

Mindful Walking

- Take a leisurely walk, whether it's indoors or outdoors
- Feel the sensation of each step—the weight shifting from one foot to the other, the ground beneath your feet
- Notice the sights, sounds, and smells around you as you walk
- Allow your mind to be present in this simple act of movement

Mindful Appreciation

- Each day, identify three things you're grateful for
- Reflect on why you're grateful for them and let that appreciation fill your heart
- It could be as simple as the warmth of the sun or a kind gesture from a colleague

Mindful Breathing

- Find a quiet spot, sit, or stand comfortably
- Close your eyes or keep a soft gaze
- Focus your attention on your breath—how it feels as it enters and leaves your nostrils or how your chest rises and falls
- If your mind wanders, gently guide your focus back to your breath

- Start with 5 minutes and gradually increase the duration

Mindfulness is a universally beneficial practice, accessible to people of all ages, backgrounds, and walks of life. Its inclusive nature allows it to cater to a diverse range of individuals, each reaping unique advantages from its practice. From stressed professionals, students, parents, and athletes to individuals seeking guidance and dealing with anxiety and other mental health conditions can use mindfulness as a complementary approach to traditional therapies.

Mindfulness is a gift that has the potential to touch the lives of countless individuals, offering a path to finding peace, resilience, and happiness within themselves and the world around them. It's an invitation to experience life fully, in all its beauty and complexity.

This book is a product of my experience in the field of beauty and wellness. I have enjoyed putting together recipes, hacks, and DIYs for the readers. I do hope that you will enjoy reading this book as much as I enjoyed writing it.

Acknowledgements

I want to express my gratitude to Chaithanya Srambickal and Pooja Verma for their help, and to Sangeeta Jain for editing the book.

By the Same Author

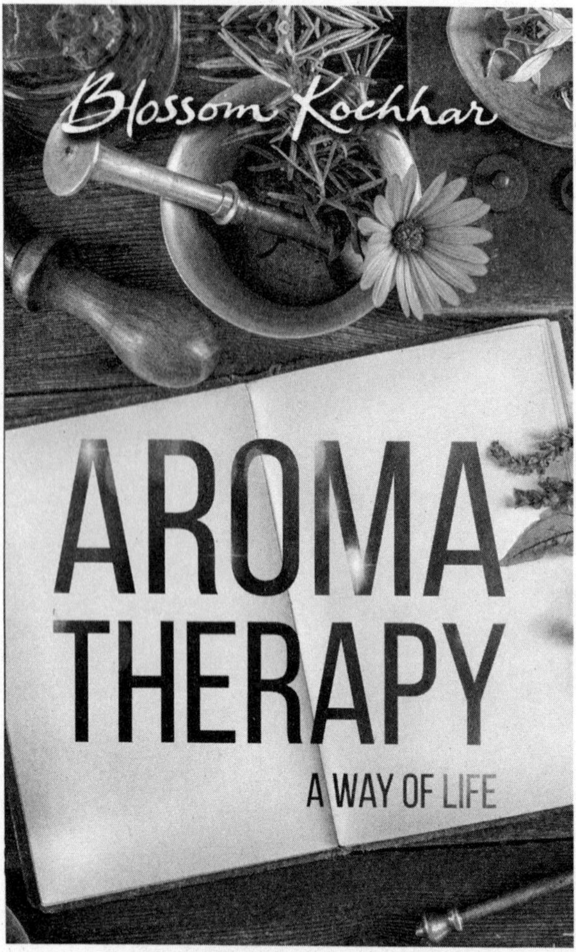